Contents

About the contributors 5

Editorial
          Dr Marie Diggins 17

Guest editorial
          Dr Adrian Falkov 21

Personal experiences 27

Chapter 1   **Messages for practice from young carers**
                  Darcey, Jamie B, Aaron, Katie, Jamie G, Abbie, Jegir, Mickela and Ste 29

Chapter 2   **Monica's story**
                  Monica Kizza... 33

Chapter 3   **Working with mentally ill parents and their families as an adult psychiatrist**
                  Professor Eleni Palazidou 35

Chapter 4   **A personal reflection on working with parents with mental ill health: obstacles and opportunities for delivering best practice**
                  Dr Joanna Fox 41

Chapter 5   **Using the Family Model in training: a light bulb moment**
                  Daphne McKenna 45

Policy and drivers for change 49

Chapter 6   **Do recent policy and legislative changes in health and social care help develop the Think Family agenda in parental mental health and child welfare?**
                  Hugh Constant 51

Chapter 7   **A change in the law doesn't always mean a change in real lives: making whole family approaches a reality**
                  Dr Moira Fraser 55

Chapter 8	What has happened to 'Think Family': challenges and achievements in implementing family inclusive practice
	Dr Jerry Tew, Professor Kate Morris, Professor Sue White, Professor Brid Featherstone and Sarah-Jane Fenton 59

Children and early intervention 65

Chapter 9	Children should be seen and heard in adult mental health services
	Ragni Whitlock and Dr Estelle Rapsey 67
Chapter 10	Early intervention to promote mental health and well-being in schools
	Dr Jane Akister and Hannah Guest 71
Chapter 11	School children's vulnerability audit tool
	Wendy Weal 75

Impacts and influences on mental health recovery, parenting and children's development and well-being 77

Chapter 12	Parental mental health and young carers: children (and families) first
	Professor Jo Aldridge 79
Chapter 13	Fathers with mental health problems: challenging stigma, promoting inclusion
	Rhys Price-Robertson and Associate Professor Andrea Reupert 83

Conceptual models 89

Chapter 14	Learning from success: conceptual introduction
	Professor Shula Ramon 91
Chapter 15	The added value of learning from success in parental mental health and child welfare work
	Dr Marie Diggins 97
Chapter 16	Success in safeguarding children in the UK
	Andy Quin 107
Chapter 17	The Family Model
	Dr Adrian Falkov 113

Assessment and interventions 121

Chapter 18 Emotional neglect, system failure and the Early Years Parenting Unit
Minna Daum and Dr Duncan McLean 123

Chapter 19 The Social Work for Better Mental Health adult mental health initiative
Dr Ruth Allen, Dr Sarah Carr and Dr Karen Linde 127

Working together 133

Chapter 20 Co-work: working in pairs enables effective whole family sessions
Dr Frank Burbach 135

Chapter 21 Keeping the family in mind: working together in Liverpool to implement a programme of innovation and change
Louise Wardale 141

Chapter 22 Think Family, Northern Ireland
Mary Donaghy 147

Research digest 153

Useful tools and resources 159

About the contributors

Dr Marie Diggins is a registered social worker. After qualifying in 1989, Marie worked for the London Borough of Lewisham and South London and Maudsley Mental Health NHS Trust until 2002. During this period Marie held a variety of positions including generic social worker, specialist mental health practitioner and, between 1995 and 2002, mental health integrated services manager.

In 2002 Marie joined the Social Care Institute for Excellence (SCIE) where she worked with key stakeholders (government departments, health and social care staff, academics and service users and carers) to identify innovative approaches to embedding evidence about what works in health and social care in different practice settings. She made particular contributions to SCIE's mental health strategy and resources, including *Think Child, Think Parent, Think Family: A guide to parental mental health and child welfare*. She was involved with SCIE's digital production since its inception in 2007 and is experienced in the development of content for eLearning, film and other digital products. Marie contributed to *Integration step by step*, SCIE's digital resource to support integrated working, drawing on her understanding of practice development, practice contexts and multi-disciplinary working environments.

While at SCIE, Marie initiated her PhD *'What works: Researching success in parental mental health and child welfare work'*, which she completed in September 2014. Marie left SCIE in 2014 and is now working independently as a part-time freelance consultant.

Dr Adrian Falkov is a senior staff specialist in child and adolescent psychiatry at Westmead (Redbank House) and Royal North Shore Hospitals in Sydney, Australia. After completing undergraduate studies in South Africa, he trained and worked in London (Guys, St Thomas' & Maudsley Hospitals) before moving to Sydney.

He is a full time clinician with longstanding interests in the impact of parental mental illness on children, family mental health, service development and evaluation (links between adult & children's mental health services) and the interface between policy and practice.

These interests have informed family focused work in mental health services using The Family Model (www.thefamilymodel.com). This approach supports greater collaboration between services to improve partnership working between clinicians, carers, consumers and their families.

The Family Model has been used in policy development, workforce capacity building and clinical work in England, Europe and Australia to improve family-focused practice in mental health services.

About the contributors

Dr Jane Akister is a reader in social work at Anglia Ruskin University, co-editor of *Practice: Social Work in Action*, and an associate mental health act manager (Cambridgeshire and Peterborough Foundation Trust). Jane's research interests include family functioning, attachment relationships and parenting support.

Professor Jo Aldridge is professor of social policy in the department of social sciences at Loughborough University, and is director of the Young Carers Research Group. She conducted the first ever study in the UK on the experiences and needs of children who live with and care for parents with serious mental health problems and she has published widely in the field of young carers and parental mental health and child welfare. Jo is also a National Institute for Health and Care Excellence Fellow.

Dr Ruth Allen is director of social work and honorary senior research fellow at South West London and St George's Mental Health NHS Trust and St George's University of London. She is a registered social worker who has worked since 1994 in mental health, in a variety of NHS and local authority organisations. She has had national leadership roles within the Social Care Strategic Network for Mental Health, the College of Social Work and is currently co-chair of the practice reference group for the chief social worker for Adults in England. In 2014 she authored the national guidance document *The Role of the Social Worker in Adults Mental Health Services*, and in 2015 co-authored three resources to implement the source guidance and develop mental health social workers' use of direct service user and family feedback to improve practice. Her research interests are domestic violence and mental health, personality disorder and the response of children's and mental health social workers, and the extension of personal health budgets in mental health.

Kate Asaf has been a childcare professional for more than 15 years. For 12 years she worked as a learning and behaviour mentor within primary education, which involved supporting children and their families to overcome a range of educational, social and personal barriers to learning. Kate is also the director of Rocks and Pebbles Ltd, an organisation that provides wrap-around childcare in a number of primary schools throughout the London Borough of Lewisham. Through her roles and interactions with children, young adults and their families, Kate has supported a large number of individuals with mental health needs as well as supported individuals to understand mental health within their homes.

Claire Barcham is a social worker and approved mental health professional (AMHP) with more than 20 years' experience in front line practice. She has worked on both local and national levels promoting excellent social work across all ages, and she currently manages a generic out of hours social work team. Claire has maintained a special interest in the interface between adults and children's work, and provides training around the law in this regard. She is also the author of the successful *The Pocketbook Guide to Mental Health Act Assessments*.

Carol Bernard is an RMN by profession and currently works as the director of commissioning for Mersey Care, and was previously the director of mental health services in Liverpool at Mersey Care NHS Trust. Mersey Care Trust provides specialist mental health and learning disability services for the people of Liverpool, Sefton and Kirkby. It has a wider role too, offering medium secure services for Merseyside and Cheshire, and high secure services covering England and Wales. The Trust campaigns for better understanding, resources and the need to challenge the stigma attached to mental distress. Carol is also the women's lead for the Trust and leads on the development of the 'Think Family' agenda, most notably the development of the Family Rooms.

Dr Frank Burbach is a consultant clinical psychologist with the Somerset Partnership NHS Foundation Trust. He is the head of clinical psychology & psychological therapies services, operational manager for the Carers and Aspergers services and lead for the Triangle of Care and Early Intervention in Psychosis. He has a diploma in marital and family therapy and is also a registered cognitive-behavioural psychotherapist. He is a member of the Triangle of Care national steering group, is the South West early intervention lead and is also a member of the editorial board of the *Journal of Family Therapy*. Dr Burbach has a PhD from Plymouth University on developing systemically-oriented mental health services and has published numerous papers and book chapters describing the development of family inclusive practice and specialist family interventions in Somerset since 1995.

Dr Sarah Carr is an associate professor of mental health research, Middlesex University, and an independent mental health and social care consultant and researcher. Sarah previously worked for the Social Care Institute of Excellence (SCIE) as a senior research analyst, where she led on a five-year Department of Health funded improvement programme on personalisation and person-centred practice. She has worked in research, information and service development roles at the National Institute for Social Work, Oxleas NHS Trust and the Centre for Mental Health. Sarah is co-chair of the National Survivor User Network (NSUN), a member of the Care Quality Commission Adult Social Care Co-production Group and is on the editorial board of *Disability and Society*. She is honorary senior lecturer at the school for social policy, Birmingham University, and visiting fellow at the school of social policy and social work at the University of York. In 2012, Sarah co-edited the book *Social Care, Service Users and User Involvement* with Professor Peter Beresford of Brunel University. Sarah has a particular interest in service user involvement and co-production, personalisation and person-centred practice and equality and diversity. She uses her lived experience of mental distress and service use in all her work.

About the contributors

Hugh Constant is a practice development manager at the Social Care Institute for Excellence (SCIE). He has worked in social care since 1993, and has practiced in residential, day care and outreach settings. He qualified as a social worker in 1997, working in the London Borough of Barnet with adults with learning disabilities before going on to manage a learning disability social work service in the London Borough of Tower Hamlets for six years. Here he led a major programme of change, focusing on improving practice and outcomes and leading a successful integration with NHS colleagues. From Tower Hamlets, Hugh joined SCIE. He led on several large projects, all focused on changing ways of working for the better in social care. He supported six local authorities across England and Northern Ireland to develop whole-family working with parents with mental health problems. He developed guidance and e-learning on assessment and eligibility, and on adult safeguarding. Hugh also worked extensively on advice and information services aimed at the general population.

Minna Daum, BA, BSc (Hons), has been practicing as a systemic family therapist since 1992. For most of that time she has specialised in carrying out and supervising multi-disciplinary court assessments and providing expert opinion on the risk of rehabilitation following abuse. In conjunction with Dr Duncan McLean, she has developed a Court Assessment Service specialising in families involving parents with personality disorders. In 2011 she and Dr McLean set up the Early Years Parenting Unit, an innovative assessment and treatment service for parents with personality difficulties and their under-five children. She has been employed as both senior family therapist and clinical manager at the Anna Freud Centre since 1998.

Mary Donaghy qualified as a social worker in 1983. Over the past 30 years, her experience has covered family and child care services (Residential & Fieldwork), children's disability services, and child and adolescent mental health services. Mary joined the health and social care board as a senior manager in 2009 to lead the regional 'Think Child, Think Parent, Think Family' project for three years. Northern Ireland was one of six national projects under the direction of the Social Care Institute for Excellence (SCIE). The project focused on improving collaborative working and enhancing a better understanding of multi-disciplinary roles and responsibilities of all stakeholders working across the adult mental health and children's services interface. Since 2012 Mary has been a social care commissioning lead for adult mental health and learning disability at the Health and Social Care Board, and she continues as regional lead for Think Family Northern Ireland. Think Family NI is now the core business of the Health & Social Care Board under the structure of Children and Young Peoples Strategic Partnership (CYPSP).

Professor Brigid Featherstone is professor of social work at the University of Huddersfield. She has researched in the areas of gender relations, fathers and family support. Her current research projects are concerned with exploring the relationship with poverty, inequality and child protection and families' perspectives on multiple services.

Sarah-Jane Fenton is a PhD student with the University of Birmingham (UK) and the University of Melbourne (Australia). Her PhD research looks at mental health services and policy for 16–25 year olds in Australia and the UK. Sarah-Jane also works as a research fellow in the Family Potential Research Centre based at the University of Birmingham. Her research interests are social policy, youth, adolescence, health policy, mental health and whole family approaches.

Dr Joanna Fox is senior lecturer at Anglia Ruskin University and her role encompasses being an academic and a researcher. Her mental health experiences are at the centre of her teaching and research interests, combined with an interest in increasing service user involvement in all aspects of mental health care and support. Joanna's own experiences inform much of her writing and research as she explores the difficulties that can be met by someone who occupies a number of different identities.

Dr Moira Fraser joined Carers Trust (formerly The Princess Royal Trust for Carers and Crossroads Care) in September 2010 as director of policy and research. She works closely with the Carers Trust network of over 160 independently managed carers centres and schemes across the UK to ensure high quality innovative local support for carers. She has been closely involved in lobbying for improved carers' rights under the Care Act, and was chair of the National Young Carers Coalition from 2012-2014, securing a landmark amendment to the Children and Families Act, recognising young carers' rights for the first time. Moira has worked in policy and campaigning work in charities for 13 years and had previously worked at Mind, the Mental Health Foundation and RNIB.

Dr Michael Göpfert grew up in Munich and trained in nursing and medicine in Germany. He completed his psychiatric and psychotherapy training in the UK and Canada and has studied parents with mental health issues and their families since 1981. He worked as a child psychiatrist and medical adult psychotherapist specialising in complex mental health needs of clients. He was very involved in medical education at the University of Liverpool, as trainer in the psychotherapies with the universities of Liverpool and Manchester and with the Royal College of Psychiatrists. He served as visiting professor in the United Arab Emirates. He worked for the General Medical Council as assessor and supervisor for doctors. Following the first publication of *Parental Psychiatric Disorder* in 1996 he was involved in major policy initiatives on parental mental health, including with the UK Social Care Institute of Excellence. Publications range from family mental health care to forensic psychotherapy. A recent award-winning initiative involved parents with complex personality issues and their children presenting at child mental health services. For many years he was involved in the care of a relative with mental health needs and he always aims to improve the lives of those with mental health issues and their families.

About the contributors

Hannah Guest was a social work student on the masters programme at Anglia Ruskin University and is now working within a statutory adult learning disability team within East Cambridgeshire as a registered social worker.

Dr Stephen Hopkins is the owner and chief executive of Touchstone Development Ltd, an education consultancy based in Lincoln, UK. Stephen has worked as a headteacher, a school inspector, a principal lecturer in a university college, and as a regional advisor for a government agency linked to change management and the reform of children's services in the UK. He has undertaken consultancy work and leadership development work for a range of public and private organisations. Dr Hopkins has an MSc from the University of East Anglia and a PhD from the University of Liverpool. He is the chair of governors of an academy, a trustee of a large academy chain, and a national leader of governance. Stephen in committed to the pursuit of social justice through high-quality education and children services and has extensive experience of working with vulnerable children and families.

Dr Karen Linde has held senior appointments in academic and development contexts with responsibility for the design of large scale change initiatives, leadership, evaluation and research activities. She has carried out innovative research in the areas of social identity, team working, the implementation of psychosocial interventions, and of systems approaches. Karen has a strong interest in the impact of organisations on the psychological health and resilience of staff and a continuing development role in the area of inequalities, with a focus on improving organisational responses to trauma, violence and abuse, and working effectively with communities in conflict.

Associate Professor Darryl Maybery from Monash University has over 70 journal publications and research grants totaling AUD3 million. His research focuses upon vulnerable families, particularly with regard to the impact of parental mental health problems on children. The central aim is to reduce the cycle of mental illness in families. In 2013, his research group were successful in obtaining a AUD1,855,891 grant to undertake the four year project 'Developing an Australian-first recovery model of parents in Victoria mental health and family services'. This program of research extends and rigorously trials the Finnish 'Lets Talk about Children' model in the family/community, adult mental health and rehabilitation sectors across Victoria. Darryl teaches in the area of research methodology and statistics and has a special teaching interest in program evaluation. Darryl was raised on a farm near Mount Arapiles in the Wimmera (Victoria, Australia) and lives in Gippsland with his partner (Andrea) and two teenage girls.

Chris McCree is a nurse with extensive experience in mental health and learning disabilities over 35 years. Her main role now is borough lead for safeguarding children in adult mental health and the lead adviser on parental mental health to children's services. This is a joint funded role between the London Borough of Southwark and South London and Maudsley NHS Foundation Trust (SLaM). Chris is a member of the Southwark Safeguarding Children Board (SSCB) and of the borough multi-agency risk assessment committee (MARAC). She is the service lead for the Southwark 'Mental Health Think Family Strategy' and is the service manager for the local authority funded parental mental health team that works with parents experiencing a range of mental health problems and who have children under five. As part of her role she provides supervision to a wide range of health and social care professionals; building and maintaining relationships across the multiagency system; providing consultation and advice. Chris has wide ranging experience as an investigator into serious incidents, both within SLaM and externally.

Daphne McKenna is an established multi-agency trainer with a proven commitment to effective collaborative working, having co-authored the SCIE parental mental health and child welfare guidance (*Think Child, Think Parent, Think Family*) and also their adult safeguarding e-learning materials. She has a proven track record as manager and child protection co-ordinator and uses these skills to raise practice standards in the delivery of training for the benefit of children and their families. She has worked extensively in the statutory sector and has more recently developed expertise in safeguarding training within the third sector.

Dr Duncan McLean is consultant psychiatrist in psychotherapy and adult and child psychoanalyst. He currently works part time at the Anna Freud Centre running a court assessment service for families with a child on the edge of care, and also runs a day unit for families and their under five children where a parent has personality difficulties.

Professor Kate Morris is a qualified social worker who joined the University of Sheffield in 2015. Before this appointment, Kate worked at the University of Nottingham (from 2009) and as the head of social work at the University of Birmingham. She gained substantial experience in practice, management and policy development before moving into social work education. Her areas of interest are family minded policy and practice, prevention, family participation in care and protection, families with complex and multiple needs and the role of social work education in promoting best practice. Kate was funded to explore the involvement of families in the reviews of cases when a child has died or suffered serious injury as a result of abuse (www.baspcan.org.uk) and is leading an exploratory study of the lived experiences of families with multiple and complex needs. This builds on her previous work for the UK government as part of the 'Think Family' policy stream, and her work internationally reviewing the evidence concerned with the impact and effect of family decision making in care and protection. Kate's current projects include an ESRC seminar series, a NORFACE grant to develop an international study of families in social work and a Nuffield project examining child welfare inequalities. Kate currently supervises PhD students in the areas of family caring relationships, family interventions in drug and alcohol and early intervention. She is active in national social work developments, is chair of JUCSWEC, and sits on the professional assembly for the College of Social Work. Kate also sits on the editorial board for the journal *Families, Societies and Relationships* and is chair of TCSW knowledge and research exchange group.

Professor Eleni Palazidou trained in psychiatry at the Joint Maudsley/Bethlem Hospitals and gained research experience at the Institute of Psychiatry where she completed her PhD in psychopharmacology awarded by the University of London. Eleni is a member of the Royal College of Physicians and the Royal College of Psychiatrists and was awarded a Fellowship of the RCPSYCH. She was an NHS University Hospital consultant psychiatrist in East London for over 20 years and is currently working as an independent consultant psychiatrist. Eleni also works as an expert witness and is listed on the UK Register of Expert Witnesses. She has widely published original research as well as chapters and books and she is on the editorial board of the *British Journal of Psychiatry-International* and other international medical journals. Her clinical and research interests have been in mood disorders, psychopharmacology and global health. She also has a special interest in parental mental health and child welfare and does assessments on parental mental health in family law cases. She is also interested in ethnic minority issues relevant to mental health.

Rhys Price-Robertson is a PhD candidate at Monash University, where he is investigating the experiences of families affected by paternal mental illness. His most recent published research has focused on fatherhood, family relationships, masculinities and child protection. Previously he worked as a researcher at the Australian Institute of Family Studies, and as a nurse in the aged care and mental health sectors. While completing a Masters of Bioethics at Monash University he was awarded the Monash-WHO Bioethics Fellowship, which saw him work as an intern in the ethics and health department of the World Health Organization in Geneva.

Andy Quin qualified as a social worker in 1981, initially specialising in work with children and families, and held team manager, middle and senior manager roles in local authority social services. Since 2007, Andy has worked independently as a social work consultant. His work for many different local authority clients has included safeguarding improvement projects, adoption panel chairing, inquiry authorship and mentoring. Andy's PhD topic concerns success and collaboration in safeguarding work and his first supervisor is Professor Ramon.

Professor Shula Ramon is the recovery research lead in the school of health and social work at the University of Hertfordshire. A social worker and clinical psychologist by training, she has been applying participatory action research in her work on mental health recovery, domestic violence, LGBT and service user involvement in social work and mental health research. Learning from success is an integral key theme in both areas of her research, as well as in her PhD supervision work. She has published 12 books and more than 100 articles in peer-reviewed journals.

Dr Estelle Rapsey is a clinical psychologist working in Somerset Partnership Adult Mental Health Services with a specialist interest in working with families. Prior to her current role, Estelle worked with young people in the Somerset Early Intervention in Psychosis Team and, in an educational setting, liaising between young people, their families and schools.

Andrea Reupert is an associate professor at Monash University, Clayton, Australia, and director of psychology programs at the Krongold Centre. Her area of expertise is in vulnerable families and developing evidence-based interventions that support families through adversity. Her team is also actively involved in developing psychosocial resources for clinicians in collaboration with people in recovery. She is the editor in chief of the journal *Advances in Mental Health*, associate editor for *Australian Psychologist*, and has served as guest editor for the *Medical Journal of Australia*. Andrea is also the co-editor for an online resource, *Gateway to Evidence that MatterS (GEMS)*, that aims to disseminate research in accessible ways to consumers, carers and clinicians. She recently co-edited a third edition of the seminal *Parental Psychiatric Disorder: Distressed parents and their families*. She has received funding from various philanthropic and governmental agencies for family-centred, inclusive approaches within an interdisciplinary and inter-agency approach.

Paul David Spencer Ross is a senior information specialist within the Social Care Institute for Excellence (SCIE), which hosts the NICE Collaborating Centre for Social Care. Paul is a chartered member of the Chartered Institute of Library and Information Professionals and has worked on a variety of topics across the social care sector. He specialises in community facilitation and knowledge growth through information and resource forums for minority and unheard groups, along with practical training in searching skills for social care research evidence.

Professor Nicky Stanley is professor of social work at the University of Central Lancashire, UK. She researches on parents' mental health, child protection, suicide and domestic violence. She has led numerous international and national research studies and is currently working on the ESMI study, which is examining the effectiveness and cost-effectiveness of perinatal psychiatry services. She contributed to the SCIE review on parental mental health and child welfare and has published papers and a book on mothers' mental health needs.

About the contributors

Dr Jerry Tew is reader in social work and mental health at the University of Birmingham and is the director of the Family Potential Research Centre – a collaboration between the University of Birmingham, the University of Nottingham and the Open University. He is an editorial board member of the *British Journal of Social Work*. His professional background is as a mental health social worker and he co-founded the Social Perspectives Network. He is currently involved in national research projects on recovery and on personalisation in mental health, and has led a national study evaluating 'whole-family' approaches in mental health. He is currently co-ordinating an ESRC funded programme of knowledge exchange around 'Family inclusive policy and practice after 'Think Family'' with a broad range of local authority, NHS and voluntary sector partners. His recent book, *Social Approaches to Mental Distress* (Palgrave Macmillan), offers an analysis of the crucial role played by social factors and life events in bringing on (or averting) mental distress, and sets out a vision for mental health practice that emphasises the centrality of issues of social identity, participation and relationship. His latest book, co-authored with Professor Jon Glasby, is entitled *Mental Health Policy and Practice* (Palgrave Macmillan), is due for publication in 2015.

Louise Wardale is a registered social worker with 27 years' experience and is Keeping the Family in Mind co-ordinator at Barnardo's. Her experience has included residential, field work, community development and strategic work across adults and children's, voluntary and statutory systems. Louise has worked as a senior practitioner in social work with Barnardo's Action with Young Carers Liverpool and for the past 13 years as the co-ordinator of an implementation plan for children and families affected by parental mental ill-health – 'Keeping the Family in Mind'. Grounded in the direct experiences of children and young people caring for and impacted by their parents' mental health problems, Louise works strategically to influence change across national and local systems, and across child and adult services. She was an active member of the Parental Mental Health and Child Welfare steering group, and a guest contributor to the SCIE guide, *Think Child, Think Parent, Think Family*. Louise is well known for the development of a range of resources, including the development of family rooms across in patient units and training materials produced in partnership with children, young people and families.

Wendy Weal is the managing director of Interface Enterprises Ltd, a national provider of specialist expertise, support and training to transform the lives of vulnerable families. Interface are a national body of expertise on effective approaches to support vulnerable families. They help local authorities and their partners jointly plan, design, implement, improve and evaluate services across priority areas relating to the needs of vulnerable families. Wendy was the deputy delivery manager of the families at risk division of the Department for Education. She had a national role in supporting local authorities and their partners in setting up and running intensive family support services for families with multiple problems, parenting support and wider reforms around integrated services and 'Thinking Family'. Wendy was the national delivery lead for the Family Pathfinders and worked with other government departments and organisations to encourage and shape a 'Think Family' approach. Examples include guidance on the development of local protocols between drug and alcohol treatment services, safeguarding boards and children and family services, offender management services, mental health services and young carers.

Professor Martin Webber is a professor of social work at the University of York. He is a registered social worker with experience of working with adults with a learning disability and mental health problems. He is passionate about achieving social change through high quality social work and social care practice with vulnerable and marginalised people. His primary research interest is the development and evaluation of social interventions with people with mental health problems. This includes primary epidemiological or methodological work, ethnographic work to develop intervention models, and experimental work to evaluate the effectiveness of interventions. He collaborates with health economists, psychiatrists, psychologists and other health scientists to maximise the effectiveness of his research. He leads the International Centre for Mental Health Social Research and also has a growing number of PhD students who are working on empirical studies in social work. He has published over 50 peer-reviewed papers and book chapters, and is an author/editor of three books. His teaching interests are in mental health social work, research methodology and the practice implications of his research. He is currently leading a team of academics from the University of York and University of Central Lancashire, under a contract from Think Ahead, to develop and deliver a new social work programme for people with an interest in working in mental health services. At the heart of this programme is training to deliver evidence-informed social interventions, which brings his research and teaching interests together.

Professor Sue White is professor of social work (children and families) at the Institute of Applied Social Studies, University of Birmingham. She researches decision making in everyday practice and how social workers and other professionals make use of moral judgements and various forms of knowledge in their work. She is also concerned with the design of organisational systems and technologies and their relation to professional sense-making.

Ragni Whitlock holds the role of clinical lead for family therapy and family-inclusive practice in Somerset Partnership Foundation NHS Trust. While her role is currently based within the adult mental health service, she has previous experience of delivering family therapy in child and adolescent inpatient and community mental health services for a number of South West NHS trusts and running a small private practice in family and couples therapy.

Editorial

Dr Marie Diggins

This book forms the first volume of Pavilion's new series of annuals, which act as a yearly update on key research, policy developments and practice innovations in the UK and elsewhere.

The literature about parental mental health and child welfare spans several decades. Research has established the potential adverse impact of adult mental illness on parenting, the parent-child relationship, the child and other family members, and the extent to which this poses a public health challenge. Problems with how adult and children's services understand and deliver support to parents with mental health problems, their children and whole families have also been identified. In contrast, far less is known about how parents with mental health difficulties and their children can be successfully supported.

In this volume and subsequent volumes, our aim is to begin to address this gap in the evidence by exploring and sharing ideas about 'success' and what 'leads to success' from the literature and from the different perspectives of parents, children and the professionals that work with them, including addressing any tensions that arise from these different perspectives.

Parents with mental health problems and their children can find it difficult to get help in an acceptable, accessible and effective manner. While not all children who have a parent with a mental health problem will be impacted negatively, there is a large and increasing body of research that highlights that many will be, and the potential of such an impact where it occurs, as well as the needs of adults with mental health problems in regard to their parenting (Webster, 1992; Stiffman *et al*, 1988; Hugman & Phillips, 1993; Cox, 1987; Darton *et al*, 1994; Cleaver *et al*, 2012).

Professionals have expressed their concerns at the barriers that get in the way of their attempts to support individuals and families successfully. These include having to work to separate and often conflicting adult and children's policy imperatives, separate training and practice guidance for adult and children's workers, services that are structured around either the adult with the mental health problem or the child, year-on-year financial cuts leading to reduced resources and frequent service re-organisation, and all of this happening at the same time as demand for services and public and government expectations are steadily increasing (SCIE, 2009; Tunnard, 2004; Diggins, 2014).

Working in either adult mental health or children and family services can be challenging. Both areas are highly emotive – they attract high levels of media attention and criticism when things go wrong, and staff can be wary of stepping outside of professional boundaries. Breaking down these professional barriers has become as important as addressing the stigma that exists in accessing services for parents and children. It has become custom and practice to talk about barriers to successful practice, rather than exploring what happens when families are supported successfully.

This annual represents a unique opportunity to address the gap in the evidence base about 'what works' by drawing together a blend of researchers, policy makers, practitioners and service users to identify both the opportunities and challenges as well as explore what works in which contexts, for whom and why. It is concerned with outcomes for parents, children and other family members as well as multi-agency staff and organisations. Contributions cover adult and children's social work and social care, adult mental health and child and adolescent mental health, carers and young carers, education, training and workforce development from all sectors. The book looks beyond the UK and presents international evidence of incidence and experience.

The policy and practice context for parental mental health and child welfare work is broad and complex as it encompasses adults and children as service users, health and social care staff from separate adult and children's services, separate adult and children's law and policy, and research that is often either adult, child or family specific.

Parental mental health and child welfare, it appears, is everybody's business. To ensure we include material that is relevant and useful to the broad range of people involved we have recruited an advisory board with considerable cross-cutting experience of research and/or delivering or receiving services. I would like to take the opportunity here to thank each of them for generously giving their time and sharing their expertise during the development of this annual.

To give a flavour of what you will find in this volume, Adrian Falkov, author of the *Family Model Handbook*, provides the guest editorial which sets out the historical context for parental mental health and child welfare work. He highlights the progress made, the challenges we still face today and how parental mental health has shown itself to be a truly global issue.

Five different personal and professional definitions of success are described in the first section. The direction of UK policy and the opportunities and challenges it presents for this area of practice are discussed in section two with contributions from SCIE, Carers Trust and Economic and Social Research Council. Three opportunities for early intervention and prevention are discussed in section three, the first in adult mental health and the second and third in schools. In section four, Jo Aldridge argues the need for professional attention on other aspects of young children's needs and young carers' lives, not just their caring role, and Andrea Reupert and Rhys Price-Robertson discuss fathers with mental illness and stigma.

A conceptual introduction to 'Learning from Success' follows in section five, followed by two examples of research that focus on learning from success; the first specific to parental mental health work and child welfare and the second to children's safeguarding. Sections six and seven incorporate a range of micro and macro interventions that have been associated with successful outcomes including the value of 'co-working', whole systems change in Liverpool and Northern Ireland, the work of the Early Years Parenting

Unit at the Anna Freud Centre and the role of mental health social work and what it has to offer parents, children, families and multi-agency colleagues.

The research digest section in this volume has been compiled by Paul David Spencer Ross from the Social Care Institute for Excellence (SCIE). A useful tools and resources section is also included.

We believe that by starting with success and focusing on different perspectives about success, this book has uncovered some new ideas about what success looks like, how it is achieved, what are the contributions and conditions most associated with successful outcomes, and why some services and professionals are beginning to overcome the barriers to success and why some cannot. Critical areas for further research and practice development are also highlighted.

References

Cleaver H, Unell I & Aldgate J (2012) *Children's Needs: Parenting capacity* (2nd edition). London: DfE; TSO.

Cox A, Puckering C, Pound A & Mills M (1987) The impact of maternal depression in young children. *Journal of Child Psychology and Psychiatry* **28** 917–928.

Darton K, Gorman J & Sayce L (1994) *Eve Fights Back*. London: MIND.

Diggins M (2014) *What Works: Researching success in parental mental health and child welfare* (PhD thesis). Anglia Ruskin University, Cambridge.

Hugman R & Phillips N (1993) Like bees round the honeypot – social work responses to parents with mental health needs. *Practice* **6** (3) pp193–205.

Social Care Institute for Excellence (2009) *Parental Mental Health and Child Welfare: Report of a practice survey* [online]. London: SCIE. Available at: www.scie.org.uk/publications/guides/guide30/files/PracticeSurvey.pdf (accessed November 2015).

Stiffman A, Jung K & Feldman R (1988) Parental mental illness, family living arrangements, and child behaviour. *Journal of Social Service Research* **11** (2/3) 21–34.

Tunnard J (2004) *Parental Mental Health Problems: Key messages from research, policy and practice*. Dartington: Research in Practice.

Webster J (1992) Split in two: experiences of the children of schizophrenic mothers. *British Journal of Social Work* **22** (3) pp309–329.

Guest editorial

Working Together: parental mental health and working with families

Dr Adrian Falkov

It is almost 50 years since Michael Rutter's Maudsley monograph, *Children of Sick Parents*, was published (Rutter, 1966); 17 years since *Crossing Bridges* (Mayes *et al*, 1998); and about eight years since the inaugural international COPMI conference in Adelaide, Australia.

Parental mental illness[1] has indeed come some considerable distance and there is now much greater awareness of the needs of parents with mental health (MH) problems and their children, a growing evidence base (Siegenthaler *et al*, 2012; Hosman *et al*, 2009; Beardslee *et al*, 2011) and a range of workforce initiatives (Reedtz *et al*, 2012; Maybery *et al*, 2012) and policies (Biebel *et al*, 2006; Solantus *et al*, 2009; State of Victoria, 2007; NSW Government, 2010).

In England, the *Think Child, Think Parent, Think Family* (SCIE, 2009) guidance has provided some support for practitioners in the field to address the mental health needs of individuals within their families, and it remains to be seen what specific impacts the recently introduced Care Act (2014), the Children & Families Act (2014) and *Closing the Gap: Priorities for essential change in mental health* (DoH, 2014) will have for this group of families (see Chapter 6).

Parental mental health (PMH) has indeed shown itself to have relevance for individuals and families, across the lifespan and generations, and across professional disciplines, service settings, agencies, localities, regions and countries – family mental health (FMH) is a truly global issue (Falkov *et al*, forthcoming).

However, progress has been slow and many barriers remain. The need for good quality information is crucial to support ongoing awareness raising and advocacy, as well as education and training to achieve the necessary acceptance, design and delivery of evidence-informed, family-focused approaches in mental health and social care services. A publication such as this one has an important role in promoting best practice and it does this by spanning the crucial gap between research and practice.

Strength in practice

A paper about eliciting positive attributes in individuals – young people in MH services (Vidal-Ribas, 2015) – recently caught my eye. It is surprising how long it has taken

---

[1] Or COPMI (Children of Parents with a Mental Illness) or FaPMI (Families with Parents experiencing Mental Illness), as the issue is known in Australia and some other parts of the world.

for the 'pursuit of resilience' (strengths-based approaches) to become accepted and incorporated into clinical practice. Clinicians will, of course, be aware of the potent validation that comes from a realistic endorsement of someone's efforts, especially in the face of adversity. We all like (and need!) praise and encouragement. My question to children, young people and their parents is: 'what gets you through?' (the bleakest, darkest times). I have yet to meet a parent, child or young person who does not struggle with this question. It sits behind the more obvious 'what are your strengths/things you are good at/successes/achievements?' (which of course those with significant adversity also struggle to answer).

I find it worth persisting and encourage exploration of both why it is a difficult question to answer and why it is such a central question to address. Of course treatment is important. But often it is controlling not curing symptoms, and the combination of good treatments (psychological, pharmacological and lifestyle) in conjunction with those innate, often hidden, qualities in the individual, is a way of tapping into a rich vein of capability that can enhance our joint efforts. It's the best form of collaboration and likely to play a considerable role in sustaining recovery and preventing relapse.

The evidence of 'lived experience'

Nowhere is this more poignantly illustrated than in the stories told by those who have lived difficult lives, shaped by illness and adversity, yet reshaped by resilience. I have known Heide Lloyd for over 15 years and we have worked together on a range of things during that time. She once again obliged when I asked if she might be interested in writing something for this inaugural annual.

Hers is a story of lifespan and generational adversity, of childhood and motherhood shaped by courage, creativity and unrelenting commitment to her children, Georgie and Hannah. Late last year she became a grandmother.

Here's what she has to say:

'Since writing my contribution to The Family Model Handbook in 2012 (Falkov, 2012), which looked at all aspects of my life with MHPs within the framework of The Family Model, life has inevitably moved forward. I am so delighted to say I have become a grandmother.

Georgie is not only a truly loving mother, she has also entered a new arena in her own life. Together we have discovered new understandings about ourselves, each other and our experiences in life.

My beautiful granddaughter, Evie, is not just the new generation – she is a wonderful little person in her own right. Some of my greatest happiness lies in the knowledge that Georgie does not judge me and my MHPs, which means that Evie and I have a wonderful bond and as much time together as I am able to cope with. I could not have anticipated how much love I would feel for my granddaughter, indeed as much as I have always felt for my own daughters. Evie has helped me rediscover that not only is love unconditional, but that where there is no love between parents with mental illness and their children, there must be acceptance, a safe home, respect at the very least. Evie is thriving in a world filled with love for her, she is safe and fascinated by everything around her.

I did not have the same parenting as Evie's mummy and daddy provide for her. As a child I learned to live inside my mind. I always hoped I gave my children a safe, happy, loving home. Well, now I know I did because my daughter has told me. It was worth the effort despite how my MHPs affected me. Now I am proud to see Georgie as a happy and besotted mother with all the usual questions that come along with a first child! I see in Evie's eyes the sincerity, purity and genuine joy of a brand new little person. I may still battle with my MHPs, but I can see what it is like not to have that struggle – and I couldn't be happier for seeing it.

Evie has, for me, reinforced a message we'd like to share – that every child needs to feel Safe and Accepted in a Family Environment while being shown (and taught how to show) Respect – SAFER. I believe it's the least we can strive to do for children despite MHPs, wherever children may be living/whomever they may be living with.'

In chapter 4 of *The Family Model Handbook* (Falkov, 2012) Heide wrote about her life:

'I first became aware that I had mental health problems when my two daughters were aged three and five. I became severely clinically depressed and was voluntarily hospitalised for nearly four months. About five months after discharge my children returned home to my full-time care.

I had postnatal depression following the birth of my first child but refused treatment, not understanding anything about mental health problems. My husband at the time had no knowledge of mental ill-health either. When I was four months pregnant with my second child my husband left me and I moved home to another area one month before her birth.

I again had postnatal depression, but did not seek help fearing that my children would be taken from me. I had no idea that treatment at that stage could have alleviated serious depressive symptoms, including obsessive suicidal thoughts, actual self-harming and continually hearing voices. It was not until I realised that I had become too ill to function as a mother that I agreed, via my GP, to a psychiatric assessment. However, my appointment with my consultant was too late for me and I was immediately hospitalised, voluntarily.

I now realise that I have been suffering from mental health problems since I was a child as a result of childhood abuse and neglect. I self-harmed frequently as a young child and I once tried to kill myself by eating poisonous plants. I took my first overdose of over-the-counter painkillers at age 11. I did not tell anyone what I had done, so I did intend to end my life.

Losing my elder daughter, Hannah, in the Sharm-el-Sheik bombings in 2005 was horrendous for both my younger daughter and me. We struggled with the terrible loss and we both suffered post-traumatic stress disorder (PTSD). No one locally was equipped to help either of us. I re-invented my ideals of parenting to try to support Georgie as best as I could. However, my own mental health problems were exacerbated and now became 'complicated' by childhood trauma, overwhelming grief, and what became "complicated PTSD". I had no idea why I had lost more of my capacity to cope with life until relatively recently. For me this is a long-term story of mental health problems, stretching back to my own birth; so that's 51 years now (which, incidentally, Georgie thinks is absolutely ancient – she is 21!).

Family focused practice: a global challenge

So progress is being made, albeit slowly, and there are increasing efforts to improve parental and family MH in many countries. In recognition of the global prevalence of MH issues in families, an international research coalition has been established. The last meeting took place in Italy in late May this year. The purpose is to foster collaborative research to improve the evidence base (for example, on family-focused practice (FFP)) and to establish networks of influence to support and facilitate systems change in mental health and related services. A series of papers will soon be published, two of which address these issues directly, listed below.

Given the inconsistent and disparate views about what constitutes FFP, Foster *et al* (in press) reviewed the literature and concluded that:

'FFP is everyone's responsibility, regardless of whether it is a child, youth or adult service. For child and youth mental health clinicians, the defining feature of FFP is the systematic incorporation of parent/carer mental health into a family-focused care plan. Conversely, for adult mental health clinicians, it is an acknowledgement of parenting and child and youth mental health. Importantly, FFP comprises clinicians' willingness, capacity and capability to see the relationship between the primary/referred person and their "key others".'

The second paper, titled *A systems approach to enhance global efforts to implement family focused MH interventions* (Falkov *et al*, forthcoming), tackles the need for global efforts to increase 'reach' (awareness about interactions, interplay and interventions for parents experiencing mental illness and their children), for intercountry comparisons on COPMI activities, identification of parents and children, and for development of service standards (e.g. for FFP). It highlights the need for broader systems change to achieve better outcomes for individuals and their families.

Integrated mental health and social care systems

Importantly, there is a need to recognise the role of all services, not just those in adult MH. For example, those practitioners working in child and adolescent MH (CAMH) and infant MH services will be familiar with inevitably raised rates of parental mental ill health (based on the impact of children's illness/difficulties on parents' MH), which, in turn, is an acknowledged complexity factor for symptom persistence, treatment resistance and engagement difficulties. So child, adolescent and youth MH services all have a crucial role, given the impact of children and young people's MH on parents and carers (the 'mirror' of COPMI is POCMI – parents of children with mental illness).

This also means that paediatric and primary care services are important, given that children with physical health problems, especially if chronic, can also precipitate or exacerbate mental ill health in parents/carers (Bardach *et al*, 2014). Children's social care services, by definition dealing with children in high-risk situations, also inevitably have major implications for carers (for example, child protection and the impact of loss associated with children's removal from parental care) and for staff – clinicians and managers – related to risk of harm as well as challenges of implementing earlier intervention to prevent such actions wherever possible.

A continuum of need: everyone's responsibility

There is, therefore, a continuum of need (Falkov, 2014) wherever a parent or child (or both) experience mental health problems and, by implication, there are associated opportunities for service responses – identification of parents or recognition of MH issues; assessment; support and intervention. This highlights the role that staff in all services have in delivering FFP.

The multi-faceted impacts of, and the interplay between, individual parental (or child) symptoms and relationships within a family, across multiple service settings (e.g. paediatrics IP, ED, community MH (AMH & CAMH)), is captured and summarised in *The Family Model* (Falkov, 2012), a summary of which is provided in this edition (see Chapter 17).

Conclusion

There is now a great deal of evidence to support family MH as a major public health issue that will require change at many levels to secure a broader approach to practice, and better outcomes for children of all ages and their parents/carers. The forthcoming paper on global approaches, mentioned previously, noted:

'Inevitably, creating an integrated, family focused, MH system of care requires broader reform.

This includes sustained effort on many fronts, including development and use of evidence – from quantitative population-based public health (how many families? how much impact?) to treatment and prevention (what works, for whom, and how?); to alliances and partnerships for advocacy with consumers and carers across the spectrum of health and social care agencies.

Inter country alliances and partnerships will be an important addition to existing initiatives.'

(Falkov *et al*, forthcoming)

References

Bardach N, Coker T, Zima B, Murphy M, Knapp P, Richardson LP, Edwall G & Mangione-Smith R (2014) Common and costly hospitalizations for pediatric mental health disorders. *Pediatrics* (doi:10.1542/peds.2013-3165).

Beardslee WR, Gladstone TR & O'Connor EE (2011) Transmission and prevention of mood disorders among children of affectively ill parents: a review. *Journal of the American Academy of Child and Adolescent Psychiatry* **50** (11) 1098–1109.

Biebel K, Nicholson J, Geller J & Fisher W (2006) A national survey of state mental health authority programs and policies for clients who are parents: a decade later. *Psychiatric Quarterly* **77** (2) 119–128.

Department of Health (2014) *Closing the Gap: Priorities for essential change in mental health* [online]. London: DoH. Available at: https://www.gov.uk/government/uploads/system/uploads/attachment_data/file/281250/Closing_the_gap_V2_-_17_Feb_2014.pdf (accessed August 2015).

Falkov A (2012) *The Family Model Handbook: An integrated approach to supporting mentally ill parents and their children.* Hove: Pavilion Publishing.

Falkov A (2014) The Continuum of Need: Parental mental health is everyone's responsibility. *Gateway to Evidence that Matters – edition 17.* Available at: http://www.copmi.net.au/images/pdf/Research/gems-edition-17-may-2014.pdf (accessed August 2015).

Falkov A, Goodyear, Hosman *et al* (forthcoming) A systems approach to enhance global efforts to implement family focused mental health (MH) interventions.

Foster K, Maybery D, Reupert A, Gladstone B, Grant A, Ruud T, Falkov A & Kowalenko N (in press) Family-focused practice in mental health care: an integrative review.

Hosman C, van Doesum K & van Santvoort F (2009) Prevention of emotional problems and psychiatric risks in children of parents with a mental illness in the Netherlands: the scientific basis to a comprehensive approach. *Australian e-Journal for the Advancement of Mental Health* **8** (3) 2250–2263.

Maybery D, Goodyear M & Reupert A (2012) The family-focused mental health practice questionnaire. *Archives of Psychiatric Nursing* **26** (2) 1–10.

Mayes K, Diggins M & Falkov A (1998) *Crossing Bridges: Training resources for working with mentally ill parents and their children – Trainer.* Hove: Pavilion Publishing.

NSW Government (2010) *Children of Parents with a Mental Illness (COPMI) Framework for Mental Health Services 2010 – 2015* [online]. Sydney: NSW Department for Health. Available at: http://www0.health.nsw.gov.au/policies/pd/2010/pdf/PD2010_037.pdf (accessed August 2015).

Reedtz C, Lauritzen C & van Doesum K (2012) Evaluating workforce developments to support children of mentally ill parents: implementing new interventions in the adult mental health care in northern Norway. *BMJ Open* **2** (3) e000709.

Rutter M (1966) *Children of Sick Parents.* Maudsley monograph. Oxford: Oxford University Press.

SCIE (2009) *Think Child, Think Parent, Think Family: A guide to parental mental health and child welfare* [online]. Available at: http://www.scie.org.uk/publications/guides/guide30/ (accessed August 2015).

Siegenthaler E, Munder T & Egger M (2012) Effect of preventive interventions in mentally ill parents on the mental health of the offspring: systematic review and meta-analysis. *Journal of the American Academy of Child and Adolescent Psychiatry* **51** (1) 8–17.

Solantus T, Paavonen EJ, Toikka S & Punamäki RL (2009) Preventive interventions in families with parental depression: children's psychosocial symptoms and prosocial behavior. *European Child and Adolescent Psychiatry* **19** (12) 883–892.

State of Victoria (2007) *Families Where a Parent has a Mental Illness (FaPMI): A service development strategy* [online]. Available at: https://www2.health.vic.gov.au/Api/downloadmedia/%7B2E6DA296-773C-455E-A278-33E14539841E%7D (accessed August 2015).

Vidal-Ribas P, Goodman R & Stringaris A (2015) Positive attributes in children and reduced risk of future psychopathology. *The British Journal of Psychiatry* **206** 17–25.

Personal experiences

Chapter 1
Messages for practice from young carers

By Darcey, Jamie B, Aaron, Katie, Jamie G, Abbie, Jegir, Mickela and Ste

Hello everyone, let's begin by introducing ourselves: we are a group of young people who are supported by Barnardo's Action with Young Carers and Young Adult Carers Service in Liverpool. We are aged between 13 and 20 years.

Did you know, one in 12 young people in every secondary school class room are young carers? A third of young carers are estimated to care for a parent with mental health problems. Did you also know, according to the latest census statistics, there are 166,363 young carers in England, compared to around 139,000 in 2001? We think there must be many more, though, and this is not the true picture.

Here in Liverpool, our city council says that there are about 5,000 young carers under 25 years old, but we know from our own experience that it's hard to come forward. But it's so worthwhile when you do, as then you really do get help and support.

We worry about our parents who we care for in case they think they are going to get in trouble. When you are a young carer like we are, it's really important that professionals work together with us and our families. We call this 'Think Family' and that means adults and children's services need to work better together. But sometimes our families are scared of the services, so that means that they might not accept help and this makes us worry more, but don't give up and please still keep trying to involve us.

First, we are children and young people who, for many reasons, have become young carers, and with our families we have been supported by Barnardo's and other services here in Liverpool. We feel that having support has helped us grow in confidence and the project has believed in us, which has made us believe in ourselves!

We wanted to share a recent presentation we did for Mersey Care NHS Trust at their annual Women and Think Family Celebration Seminar. It's not that easy standing up – bit nervy – and that's why putting it in this letter is good so more people can read it!

A number of years ago a group of young carers just like us who were supported by the service came up with 10 great messages to adult mental health professionals and this is what they said:

1. Introduce yourself. Tell us who you are and what your job is.
2. Give us as much information as you can.
3. Tell us what is wrong with our parents.
4. Tell us what is going to happen next.
5. Talk to us and listen to us. Remember, it is not hard to speak to us – we are not aliens.
6. Ask us what we know and what we think. We live with our parents. We know how they have been behaving.
7. Tell us it is not our fault. We can feel really guilty if our Mum or Dad is ill. We need to know we are not to blame.
8. Please don't ignore us. Remember we are part of the family and we live there too!
9. Keep on talking to us and keeping us informed. We need to know what is happening.
10. Tell us if there is anyone we can talk to. Maybe it could be you!

We spent time before the event planning what we wanted to say. We knew that the messages above were understood, but were they always happening? So we wanted to try a different way to get our views over! We wanted it to be lively, so we had large pieces of a jigsaw and we called out letters and asked the audience to get involved – they did! We told them that they can help join up our jigsaw and with each piece we read out our views. We had 11 pieces and this is how it went!

T stands for TRUST
As a young carer, trust is so important. We can worry about sharing things and we need to know who we can trust so they can help us. Trust is an important part of Young Carers Assessments. But we want to say that the word 'assessment' is not one that we like using – since we understand assessment to mean something that you pass or fail – in school we do controlled assessments, which are our GCSEs.

But the assessment in Barnardo's is the opportunity to share our experiences, talk about our caring roles and think about the parts of our lives we want to improve and plan together how this might happen.

H stands for HELP
Sometimes as young carers we need help because we cannot do everything. But we try our best. Maybe you might be able to help?

I stands for INDEPENDENCE
As it's only ever been me and my mum at home, I have grown up to be a very independent individual. This has helped me in a positive way as it has enabled me to open many doors. But independence doesn't mean I still don't care for my mum.

N stands for NO WRONG DOOR
Barnardo's was not the wrong door for me – but many families need help early and that means all services' doors should be open to help families like ours.

K stands for KNOWLEDGE
Being a young carer means we need an understanding of our parent's illness or disability. Knowledge of this helps us so much; we then understand that it's not our fault and this helps us to keep going when we feel low.

F stands for FAMILY
We are part of a family; we know what's going on, so please don't push us out. We may be young but we know more about our family, so 'Think Family' in all that you do, please.

A stands for ABBIE
I'm 14 and I think I started caring from about seven years old. Being a young carer is hard but can be fun at times. One day you can be living a normal child's life, then the next day you are being an adult and doing parental jobs, taking care of siblings, doing washing, making tea, sorting out medication and a lot more.

You do need support to help tackle what life throws at you. A young carer needs to have strong shoulders to carry out their role. We love our parents. We don't decide to become young carers – often you don't know you are one until you are told.

M stands for MATURITY
Not feeling like we are being taken seriously or as seriously as we want, and feeling that we are talked to as if we are kids. Professionals need to know that … we have had to grow up quickly; we can and do get stressed.

Just because we are tired in school doesn't mean that we are lazy.

Just because we do things for our parents doesn't mean that they are lazy either.

I stands for INVISIBLE and INVINCIBLE
Often, young carers are ignored by professionals. This makes them feel invisible. Young carers are not invincible – how will you notice them if you treat them as if they are invisible?

L stands for LOVE and LIFE
Sometimes it can be hard looking after your family, but I love them and they love me.

Y stands for YOU
This isn't just about us as young people and young carers. This is about you as well. Think about approaching us a family unit and not just as an individual.

So, now our jigsaw had been completed by the audience and it spelt out Think Family. We wanted them to know that we really benefit from this joined up way of working. We know lots of workers do try to make this happen, and together we can ALL make a difference — we know this first hand.

Thanks for reading this.

Kind regards

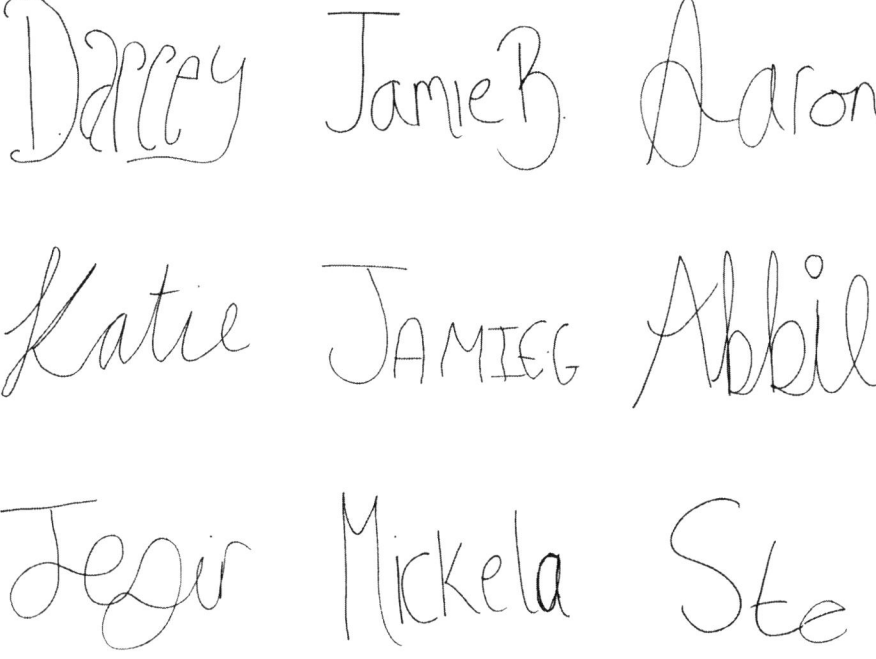

Darcey, Jamie B, Aaron, Katie, Jamie G, Abbie, Jegir, Mickela and Ste

Barnardo's Action with Young Carers and Keeping the Family in Mind Liverpool

Chapter 2
Monica's story

By Monica Kizza

Dear Reader,

My name is Monica. I am 46 years of age and a very proud and resolute single mum of three wonderful children. I would like to share my story with you and how my personal experiences have made me the woman and the mum that I am today.

I was born in Uganda and lived a happy childhood. Having had a good education, I moved into a successful career and then began to develop a business to support women's empowerment. I married in 1991, had my first daughter in 1995, and my life was looking positive, though, as I tell my story, you will read how dramatic changes occurred that have had a great impact on my whole family.

I was expecting my second child in 2001 and it was during this time that my then husband, a medical student, came over to Liverpool to study for his PhD and I remained at home in Uganda. I felt it was my duty to support him and he reassured me that by coming to Liverpool after I had our second baby I would be able to continue my education and develop the women's empowerment business I so loved.

So, a year later I arrived in Liverpool and joined him together with our six-year-old daughter and six-month-old son, believing we had a new life in front of us. I could not have predicated how my life would now take a totally different and despairing path. Before I left Uganda, we had decided to rent out our house and sold many of our belongings to finance the move and to invest in a project to sustain our financial future.

There was a requirement for him to go abroad to do a research programme, and when I joined him in Liverpool he was just about to go to Malawi. While he did leave, it was not for Malawi as he had told me, but to Uganda. It was a dramatic change of decision and by then I had just fallen pregnant with my third baby. I got to hear from family and friends that he was leaving with his mistress and had betrayed me.

Here I was with two small children in a foreign country, I had no idea of the culture, the geography of the place and how to get around, get shopping, pay bills and just get by. I was so frightened, so alone and so worried that it froze me.

I had been here for four months believing our future was hopeful and now I was on my own and my downward spiral began to take hold. I broke down, crying and crying every single night, believing there was no hope for me and my children. We had to leave the housing association property as I could not pay the rent – I had nothing. I managed to locate a church nearby that took us in and supported me through my pregnancy. Meanwhile, mail was being sent to me regarding arrears for debts that my ex-husband had accrued.

I felt so very alone, abandoned, rejected with no point in living. Yet I had two children looking to me, relying on me, and knowing I was now pregnant my world was falling apart. It was then that I was diagnosed with clinical depression.

I had a major breakdown; my GP, health visitor and the CAB all helped but I don't recall the details – for a number of years I blocked it out, I believe to somehow hold onto life. Sometime later I was then referred to a consultant psychiatrist in the local mental health trust – Mersey Care NHS Trust – and that was my saving grace. I felt they cared for me and understood that I am a human and it was ok to feel the way I did. They recognised, most importantly, that I was a mum who needed support and who deeply loved her children.

Through my Mersey Care family support worker, who was with me every step of the way, I was introduced to Barnardo's Action with Young Carers Liverpool. It was sensitively recognised that my children had been taking on so many caring responsibilities for me. I had had no choice; they had had no choice, and they were now in need of support. They had been shouldering the burden, trying so hard to keep us together, helping me to get better, and now they were breaking. I know with complete certainty that this referral to Barnardo's was a turning point in my battle with depression and getting support for my whole family. I have drawn what I call the 'Deadly Cycle', which sums up how I saw our family situation.

Monica's story

The Deadly Cycle

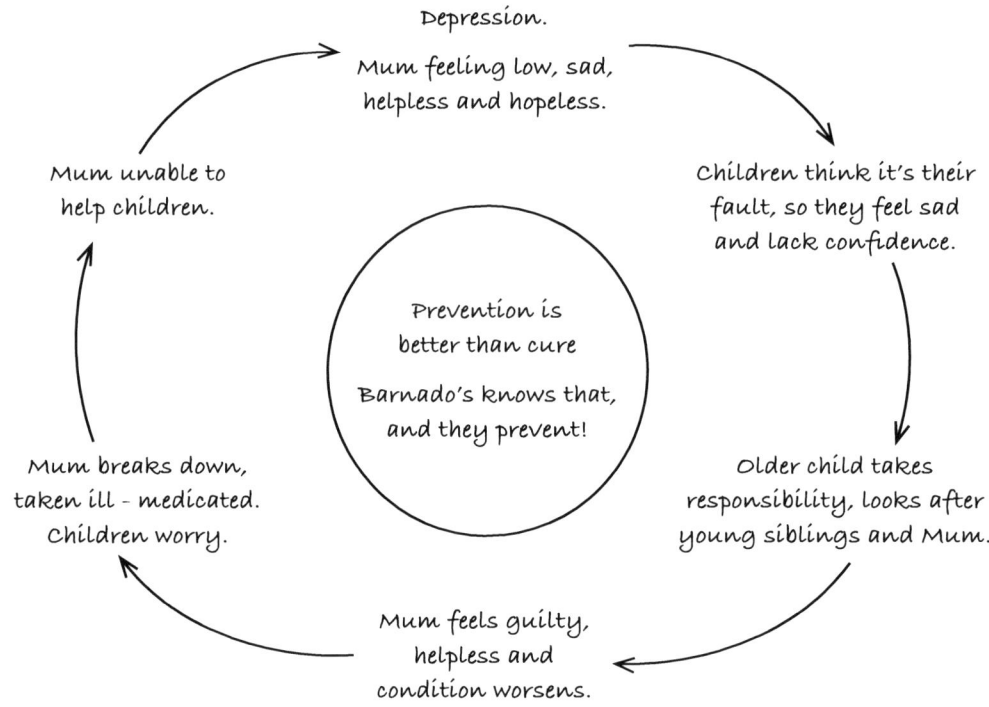

Sadly, I have suffered much stigma and lost friends due to their misunderstanding of my mental health problems. But I look for the positives: our Barnardo's young carers worker and the Trust's family support worker have shown that adult and children's services can work together so well, and they complement one another. I didn't know what a 'team around the family' was, but I soon felt that this approach was working well. My children and I are at the centre and together we work with the professionals, which has built our confidence and resilience. Of course problems still remain, but we have all gained the strength to help ourselves and move forward.

My children are growing into confident young people who, despite the negative impacts they have experienced, have been and continue to be supported. Their future, I know, is bright, and my love for them has always been paramount – the most important role I have is to be a good parent. I'm using my skills to empower others now; I am training as a counsellor and on my road to recovery.

I know our lives are turning around, I feel I have come from the ashes, rising up again, and this is attributed to the support we have around us all. I know there is hope…

Yours sincerely

Monica Kizza

Chapter 3
Working with mentally ill parents and their families as an adult psychiatrist

By Professor Eleni Palazidou

Introduction

At any given time one in six people in the UK will experience mental illness, with a lifetime morbidity of 25%. The large majority will have common disorders such as depression and anxiety and about 0.5% will have a psychotic illness (Parker & Beresford, 2008).

It is estimated that 50% to 66% of parents with a serious and enduring mental illness (mainly schizophrenia, bipolar disorder and severe depression) live with one or more children under 18. Often these children find themselves in the role of carer. According to the 1991 census, as many as 175,000 young people in the UK were caring for a parent or other family member with mental health problems. Parental mental health is often a reason for children entering the care system and a substantial percentage (about 50 to 90%) of parents on children's social workers' caseload have mental health or substance misuse problems (Dearden & Becker, 2004).

Mental illness is often associated with lower socio-economic status and has high comorbidity with substance misuse, both of which add to the burden of disease for the parents. An additional problem in some families, particularly in younger mothers, is the exposure to violence from male partners (McPherson *et al*, 2007). All these adversities, which are commonly present, complicate the life of the mentally ill and increase the burden of disease on the family as a whole. However, the most vulnerable and most affected are the children who live with the mentally ill parent (Kinsella *et al*, 1996).

Children's mental health: how can it be protected?

Not all children living with mentally ill parents will develop mental health problems themselves. However, the risk is high and one-third to two-thirds of them will experience their own mental health difficulties at some point in their life (ODPM, 2004). This occurs partly through genetic transmission and partly through environmental influences. The role of the environmental influences is complex and these include not only the direct effects of the parent's mental illness but also other people's attitudes and behaviour towards the family, associated with the stigma of mental illness. This often extends to school where the child may be subjected to teasing or bullying by other children, because of the parent's mental illness.

Although it is not possible to eliminate genetic influences, there is a lot that can be done to minimise negative environmental factors and enhance protective ones to increase resilience to mental health problems. Appropriate understanding and support in keeping with the different individual needs of all the family members is essential. Such support needs to remain in place over time and be flexible, so that it can be promptly and effectively adjusted to any changes in circumstances (Falkov, 1998).

The views of both parents and children are important in planning the necessary interventions. *Crossing Bridges* (Falkov, 1998) synthesised the findings of four separate studies (shown in boxes 1–3)

Box 1: What parents want for themselves

- ▶ More understanding and less stigma and discrimination in relation to mental health problems.
- ▶ Support in looking after their children.
- ▶ Practical support and services.
- ▶ Good quality services to meet the needs of their children.
- ▶ Parent support groups.
- ▶ Child-centred provision for children to visit them in hospital.
- ▶ Ongoing support from services beyond periods of crisis.
- ▶ Continuity in key worker support.
- ▶ Freedom from fear that children will inevitably be removed from them.

(Falkov, 1998)

Box 2: What parents want for their children

- ▶ Opportunities for children to talk about any fears, confusion and guilt.
- ▶ Opportunities for children to meet adults they can trust, and to participate in activities where they can meet other children.
- ▶ Provision of explanation and discussion about the events and circumstances surrounding the parental mental health problems.
- ▶ Continuity of care and minimal disruption of routines during a crisis (including hospitalisation of parent/carer).

(Falkov, 1998)

Box 3: What children and young people want

What children and young people want

- ▶ Age-appropriate information about the illness and prognosis.
- ▶ Someone to talk to – not necessarily formal counselling.
- ▶ A chance to make and see friends.

What children and young people taking on a caring role want

- ▶ Practical and domestic help.
- ▶ Recognition of their role in the family.
- ▶ A contact person in the event of a crisis regarding a parent.

(Falkov, 1998)

Parental mental illness and the adult psychiatrist's role

The National Confidential Inquiry into Suicide and Homicide (DCSF, 2008) reviewed 254 homicide convictions between 1997 and 2004 in England and Wales where children were killed by their biological or step parents. It was found that 37% (94 out of 254) of those convicted had a mental disorder (15% depressive disorder, 11% personality disorder, 8% schizophrenia/other delusional disorder and 5% substance misuse). The most important risks to the children identified by the inquiry were the parents' delusional beliefs involving the child or a suicide plan involving the children.

These cases are rare but psychiatrists are required to be highly alert to such risks and ensure scrupulous assessment and monitoring as appropriate. It should be noted that the large majority of mentally ill parents are not a risk to their children but they need support in order to fulfil effectively their parental role.

The Children Act (2004) identifies children whose parents suffer from mental illness as one of the key groups of vulnerable children. *Safeguarding Children: Working together under the Children Act 2004* (The Welsh Government, 2007) asks that all health professionals working with adults need to be alert to the needs of children. They should routinely enquire about any dependent children or those children with whom the adult patient has significant contact. This highlights the importance of routinely identifying and recording if adults who use mental health services are parents or carers.

Mental illness in a parent or carer does not necessarily have an adverse impact on a child, but it is always essential to assess its implications for any children involved in the family. Being a parent with a mental health need may be particularly challenging. Many parents are painfully aware that their disorder affects their children even if they do not fully understand the complexities (Falkov, 1998). The Royal College of Psychiatrists (2011) states that *'data indicate that 10–15% of children in the UK live with a parent who has a mental disorder and 28% of those are the children of lone parents with a mental disorder'*.

While the National Patient Safety Agency (2009) report *Preventing Harm to Children from Parents with Mental Health Needs* puts the emphasis on children's safety, requiring all chief executives of mental health trusts to ensure a series of actions (see box 4), the Royal College of Psychiatrists (2011) has issued a more comprehensive guidance to psychiatrists, which although it also emphasises child protection matters, it makes recommendations on supporting the mentally ill in their role as parents (see box 5).

Box 4: Actions for mental health trusts

▶ All assessment, care programme approach (CPA) monitoring, review and discharge planning documentation and procedures should prompt staff to consider if the service user is likely to have or resume contact with their own child or other children in their network of family and friends, even when the children are not living with the service user.

▶ If the service user has or may resume contact with children, this should trigger an assessment of whether there are any actual or potential risks to the children, including delusional beliefs involving them, and drawing on as many sources of information as possible, including compliance with treatment.

▶ Referrals should be made to children's social care services under local safeguarding procedures as soon as a problem, suspicion or concern about a child becomes apparent, or if the child's own needs are not being met. A referral must be made:

  ▶ if service users express delusional beliefs involving their child

  ▶ if service users might harm their child as part of a suicide plan.

▶ Staff working in mental health services should be given clear guidance on how to make such referrals, including information sharing, the role of their organisation's designated lead for child protection, and what to do when a concern becomes apparent outside normal office hours.

▶ A consultant psychiatrist should be directly involved in all clinical decision making for service users who may pose a risk to children.

▶ Safeguarding training that includes the risks posed to children from parents with delusional beliefs involving their children, or who might harm their children as part of a suicide plan, is an essential requirement for all staff. Attendance, knowledge and competency levels should be regularly audited, and any lapses urgently acted on.

(National Patient Safety Agency, 2009)

> **Box 5: Royal College of Psychologists recommendations**
>
> ▶ All psychiatrists and members of multidisciplinary teams should be familiar with legal and policy frameworks in relation to safeguarding children.
>
> ▶ Training in safeguarding is essential and attendance, knowledge and competence levels should be regularly audited; any lapses should be urgently acted on.
>
> ▶ All assessment, CPA monitoring, review and discharge planning documentation and procedures should prompt staff to consider parenting issues.
>
> ▶ Any assessment should measure the potential or actual impact of mental health on parenting. Remember the children's rights to be safeguarded are paramount, even when they are perceived as interfering with the therapeutic relationship.
>
> ▶ Referrals should be made to children's social care services under local safeguarding procedures as soon as a problem, suspicion or concern about a child becomes apparent, or if the child's own needs are not being met. Referrals must be made:
>
>   ▶ if service users express delusional beliefs involving their child
>
>   ▶ if service users might harm their child as part of a suicide plan.
>
> ▶ Be conversant with guidance on how to make referrals to children's social care services, including information sharing, the role of their organisation's designated lead for child protection, and what to do when a concern becomes apparent outside normal office hours.
>
> ▶ Consider the possibility of unplanned pregnancy and discuss contraception as well as the risk of pregnancy. Give culturally sensitive information at each stage of assessment, diagnosis, disorder course and treatment about the impact of the disorder and its treatment (including medication) on their health and the health of the foetus or child.
>
> ▶ In the community where children may be part of the household, note that the Mental Capacity Act (2005) does not have provision for the protection of others. Therefore, if an intervention is needed in individuals who are parents, partly for the protection of children, the Mental Health Act (1983) must be used (in Scotland, the Children (Scotland) Act (1995) allows the removal of an adult from the house if a child is going to come to harm at the hand of that adult). When arranging the Mental Health Act assessment, the local safeguarding team should be contacted and any relevant information sought from them.
>
> ▶ Inpatient settings should ensure that contact between parents and children when a parent is in hospital is actively encouraged and that there are family visiting rooms, which are warm, clean and well equipped.
>
> (summarised from The Royal College of Psychiatrists, 2011)

The Care Programme Approach (CPA)

Adult mental health practitioners are expected to routinely review their patients' condition (those with serious and enduring mental illness) in the context of a multidisciplinary setting. The revised version of the CPA process, 'Refocusing CPA', sets out the values and principles that underpin good practice in mental health services and considers the family as an essential part of this process.

It requires the individuals' care and support to be placed at the 'centre' and promotes social inclusion and recovery. It recognises the individual as a person first and a patient or service user second. Very importantly, the care assessment and planning views a person 'in the round'; seeing and supporting them in their individual diverse roles and the needs they have, which includes family and parenting amongst others (Department of Health, 2008).

The recently published document *Safeguarding Children Standards for Adult Mental Health* by Public Health Wales (Public Health Wales, 2015) and distributed to health boards and NHS trusts as well as the Safeguarding Children NHS Network, is a welcome contribution to the field. Its purpose is to support adult mental health services in identifying service users with a parenting or caring role and ensure appropriate professional intervention as necessary. It identifies a number of mental health standards (summarised in box 6) and the recommended actions are stated with clarity.

> **Box 6: Safeguarding Children Standards for Adult Mental Health**
>
> **Mental health standards**
>
> As part of all mental health assessments each episode of treatment whether at an inpatient unit or in the community, the mental health professionals will:
>
> ▶ Routinely record/confirm whether the adult being assessed is a parent or has a significant caring role for a child.
>
> ▶ Establish and record details of the children, the parenting arrangements and what agencies are currently involved.
>
> ▶ Following assessment, professionals should routinely inform midwifery, health visiting or school nursing services as appropriate. If the initial referral was not from the GP, primary care should be notified of any concerns that may impact upon an adult's parenting or caring capacity. Reassess at each further contact.
>
> ▶ Referral process must be followed in line with the All Wales Child Protection Procedures. Where professionals suspect a child and/or unborn child has suffered or is at risk of suffering significant harm as the result of commission or omission on the part of the parent/carer, the referral process must be followed. An appropriate child protection referral should not be delayed, for example because a diagnosis has not yet been made in relation to the adult.
>
> ▶ Professionals working within adult mental health services must ensure that their care planning includes explicit details about issues and interventions required to help their clients in their parenting role. Consideration must be given to the adults' role as a parent and the impact of their mental ill health on their parenting capacity, and subsequently on their children. This should also consider the wishes and feelings of the child regarding the parent's illness.
>
> ▶ Where there are issues about children's welfare, discharge plans must be involved and be agreed by all professionals working with the family. Discharge planning needs to be robust to ensure that the child's physical and emotional needs are met.
>
> ▶ The needs of children should be explicitly considered within the planning processes. Where there are concerns about service users' ability to care for their children due to their mental state, and following referral, children's services should be invited to attend a meeting.
>
> (Public Health Wales, 2015)

Mental illness generally presents for the first time at a young age, usually in the teenage years and early twenties. Given the chronic relapsing nature of most psychiatric conditions and the way mental health services are organized to ensure long term continuity of care, the consultant adult psychiatrist will usually be working with the individual with mental illness from early adulthood, through to parenthood. The consultant adult psychiatrist has a major role to play alongside other agencies in trying to help make this journey as smooth as possible for the mentally ill parent. A relationship of trust needs to be developed between doctor and patient in order to achieve an effective collaboration between them. In general, the patient perceives the doctor as their advocate and this is what the doctor also prefers as his or her primary role. In practice this is not always possible, as the psychiatrist often has to make decisions that go against the wishes of the patient, for example, in situations when the Mental Health Act needs to be implemented for compulsory treatment, or when there are child protection issues and possible care orders.

For all these reasons, the role of the psychiatrist in managing mental illness in parents is very complex. The traditional role of being responsible for the health and welfare of the individual patient and to 'do no harm' as far as that person is concerned are seriously challenged by the realities of parenthood. The psychiatrist is required to consider not only the health and safety of the patient under his or her care but also the health and safety of others who may be affected by the patient's mental state, and in particular the well-being of their offspring.

The existence of rules and policies imposes additional roles and responsibilities upon the psychiatrist, which conflict with the more comfortable role of the doctor as the therapist. They are expected to 'police' their patient's behaviour and report any concerns about risk to others, hence 'betraying' patient confidentiality. When shared with other agencies, this information may lead to the patient losing custody of their children, temporarily or permanently. If such situations are not handled carefully and sensitively they may cause irreparable damage to the therapeutic doctor-patient relationship. However difficult it may be, this task can be made easier if frank and sensitive discussions around parenting and children's welfare take place early on in the management of people of reproductive age, ideally before conception, and continue during the pregnancy period and after childbirth. Anticipating and dealing with problems as they arise and engaging the patient in an informed and considerate way, facilitates effective working towards prevention of crises and possible loss of custody.

Ensuring good illness control is the doctor's primary responsibility and the best prevention strategy. Psycho-education is of paramount importance. Explaining to the patient the nature of their illness and the need for ongoing medication and ensuring that any adverse effects of drug treatments are noted and dealt with effectively, goes a long way towards patient concordance and compliance with treatment. In due course, when adequate symptom control is achieved, patients become more aware of the importance of treatment and engage more effectively with their care plan. Keeping children's custody is the primary motivating factor for staying in treatment for mothers with mental illness.

Conclusion

The consultant adult psychiatrist's role is multifaceted in relation to mentally ill parents, and they need to work collaboratively with other agencies in order to achieve optimum outcomes for their patients. The involvement of the children's social services at an early stage, when they can offer the mentally ill parent support and practical assistance, rather than the threat of care orders, can have a preventive role and helps dissolve much of the fear and suspicion from the part of the sick parent. In most cases joint working between the adult mental health services, the children's social services and the mentally ill parents, with understanding, sensitivity, persistence and honesty, a supportive and problem solving approach, together with optimum treatment of the illness, may secure the much needed co-operation of the patient, and be effective in preventing long separations of children from their parents.

References

Dearden C & Becker S (2004) *Young Carers in the UK: the 2004 report* [online]. London: Carers UK and The Children's Society. Available at: http://www.lboro.ac.uk/microsites/socialsciences/ycrg/youngCarersDownload/YCReport2004%5B1%5D.pdf (accessed August 2015).

DCSF (2008) *Analysing Child Deaths and Serious Injury Through Abuse and Neglect: What can we learn?* London: Department for Children, Schools and Families.

Department of Health (2008) *Refocusing the Care Programme Approach: Policy and positive practice guidance.* London: The Stationery Office. Available at: http://webarchive.nationalarchives.gov.uk/20130107105354/http:/www.dh.gov.uk/prod_consum_dh/groups/dh_digitalassets/@dh/@en/documents/digitalasset/dh_083649.pdf (accessed October 2015).

Falkov A (Ed.) (1998) *Crossing Bridges: Training resources for working with mentally ill parents and their children – Reader for managers, practitioners and trainers.* Hove: Pavilion Publishing.

Kinsella KB, Anderson RA & Anderson WT (1996) Coping skills, strengths and needs as perceived by adult off spring and siblings of people with mental illness – a retrospective study. *Psychiatric Rehabilitation Journal* **20** (2) 24-32.

McPherson MD, Delva J & Cranford JA (2007) A longitudinal investigation of intimate partner violence among mothers with mental illness. *Psychiatric services* **58** (5) 675-680.

National Patient Safety Agency (2009) *Preventing Harm to Children from Parents with Mental Health Needs.* Available at: http://www.nrls.npsa.nhs.uk/resources/?entryid45=59898 (accessed October 2015).

NSPSA (2009) www.nspsa.nhs.uk/patientsafety/alerts-and-directive

ODPM (2004) *Mental Health and Social Exclusion: Social Exclusion Unit report* [online]. London: Office of the Deputy Prime Minister. Available at: http://tse.two-seas.eu/filelib/file/mentalhealthsocialexclusion.pdf (accessed September 2015).

Parker G & Beresford B (2008) *Protocol for SCIE Systematic Review on the Prevalence, Incidence and Detection of Parental Mental Health Problems.* York: Social Policy Research Unit: University of York.

Public Health Wales (2015) *Safeguarding Children Standards for Adult Mental Health.* Available at: http://www.rcpsych.ac.uk/pdf/Mental%20Health%20Standards%20July%202015%20%202%20(2)%20Safeguarding%20Children%20Standards%20for%20Adult%20Mental%20Health.pdf (accessed October 2015).

Royal College of Psychiatrists (2011) *CR164 Parents as Patients: Supporting the needs of patients who are parents and their children.* Available at: http://www.rcpsych.ac.uk/usefulresources/publications/collegereports/cr/cr164.aspx (accessed October 2015).

The Welsh Government (2007) *Safeguarding Children: Working together under the Children Act 2004.* Available at: http://gov.wales/topics/health/publications/socialcare/circular/nafwc1207/?lang=en (accessed October 2015).

Chapter 4

A personal reflection on working with parents with mental ill health: obstacles and opportunities for delivering best practice

By Dr Joanna Fox

Introduction

All mothers and fathers have stories of the difficulties and joys they encountered on their road to parenthood. However, many parents with a diagnosis of mental ill health have unique and poorly understood challenges (Fox, 2012). This short reflection recounts the experience of professional involvement in my life from the moment my partner and I decided to have a child. The account is told from my perspective as a person with a diagnosis of schizophrenia, although a quite different version may have been given by the professionals who cared for me.

As a mother with a diagnosis of schizophrenia, I balance a number of different valued social roles, including senior lecturer in social work, registered social worker with the Health and Care Professionals Council (HCPC), researcher, wife, and at this time, a PhD student. The overwhelming role that concerned practitioners during my journey to parenthood was that of a service user with a diagnosis of schizophrenia.

The journey of parenthood

As a person with a mental health issue, the journey to successful parenthood began long before I could contemplate having a baby. It began when I managed to recover after the catastrophic effects of mental health trauma (Anthony, 1993), and when I found the right partner and was able to explain to him that I have a diagnosis of schizophrenia. He accepted me with this diagnosis and its concomitant issues, and we got married. The next step in many couple's lives is to contemplate having a family. However, when one member of that couple has a potentially serious hereditary illness, this discussion takes on another dimension: our child could have an increased chance of developing schizophrenia.

How can professionals manage and counsel such families who have these decisions to make? My psychiatrist, whom I had known for a long time, reassured me that my life was of value, so the chances were that a child of mine would also have a good life with well-managed mental health. My husband and I took the bold decision to have a child together. This can be a difficult position for professionals: how can they manage this decision when they fear the parents' possible failure to look after their child effectively? Although this fear was not an issue in our case, professionals need to warn of the potential risks that a parent with mental ill-health might encounter but also support a parent if they decide to have a child.

The next step for us was considering whether and how much medication I should take during pregnancy. At this point I had been taking medication for 18 years and had found it very successful in managing my mental health. I decided to stop taking medication to see if I could manage without it – a decision that I relayed to the psychiatrist. I became mentally unwell after three months and decided very quickly to start taking medication again. This was a difficult experience for my husband as he watched his mentally well wife become paranoid and a little confused. This revealed some of the real experiences of mental distress that my husband had never seen before. This was a reasonable experiment but one that reinforced the need for me to continue medication.

The evidence of the safety of the atypical anti-psychotics in pregnancy is limited (Brunner *et al*, 2013; Gentile, 2010), however it was clear to me that I needed to take medication. My psychiatrist suggested that I take an older, typical anti-psychotic, which had more evidence of safety in pregnancy, however the side effects of dry mouth and increased sedation were intolerable. I therefore returned to taking olanzapine, which effectively managed my symptoms. This was a difficult decision because olanzapine causes increased hunger which leads to increased weight and increased chances of diabetes, and there is only limited data on its safety in pregnancy (Brunner *et al*, 2013).

My psychiatrist recommended that a community psychiatric nurse (CPN) monitor my mental health in the last three months of my pregnancy. He warned me that maternity staff could demonstrate quite significant concern about a mother of a young baby with a mental health problem. I agreed to this support and was allocated a very sensible and experienced CPN, who was able to advocate on my behalf. The pregnancy was managed well and I was seen by the obstetrician, who monitored my baby's health, and also by a community midwife.

At 36 weeks of pregnancy I had a shock: I received a letter from the safeguarding midwife for adults and vulnerable children inviting me to a meeting of the professionals caring for me. I was given no warning of this letter, no choice of dates, and was given no information as to the content of the meeting. I was angry and upset although my husband warned me not to be too confrontational as I would be perceived as non-compliant – not a good label to have when professionals seemingly hold all the power.

The meeting was attended by my husband and me, the community midwife, the health visitor, my CPN and the safeguarding midwife. I conveyed that the meeting was poorly organised with little information as to why it had been convened. This protest was noted. I was informed that it was advisable that I stayed in hospital for 48 hours after the birth and that my baby and I would be visited everyday by a professional for four weeks following discharge from hospital. I was advised that the birth should be obstetrician-led rather than midwife-led. I felt angry, frustrated and upset, but very powerless.

My daughter's birth was two weeks overdue so labour was induced. As no beds were available in the obstetrician-led unit, I had a midwife-led birth after all. The birth was as good as it could have been, with my husband supporting me and advocating to ensure that I had the water birth I had wanted. I then stayed in hospital for 24 hours but was discharged as the baby and I were obviously well, and, moreover, there was a shortage of maternity beds.

The midwives, community health visitors and CPN continued to visit for two weeks. We had a variety of professionals coming to visit us, but when I protested, the child development team agreed that professionals who knew me would visit me whenever possible. This was a real concession from the health visiting team and an example of good practice, although when they visited they always seemed to wake our little daughter when we had just got her to sleep. It was clear that she was thriving and putting on weight. Despite this, having a new baby can be de-skilling and disempowering as the parents are thrust into this new experience. I found that the professionals caring for me lost sight of the other identities that I had, the valued social roles, and related only to the identity that they gave me – that of service user. I had little confidence in my abilities as I felt the expectation of failure on me from the different professionals. This affected my early bonding with my daughter as I found it so hard to find the rhythm of motherhood. My husband supported me throughout and helped me to manage my frustration and lack of confidence.

Individual professionals also agreed to me visiting them at the children's centre[1] instead of visiting me at home. This was good practice and helpful in enabling me to engage as a 'normal' mother. They were reassured when I engaged with the mothers' groups at the children's centre – although I found the groups consisted of women I had little connection with.

Discussion

As I write this, my daughter is now nearly five years old – a very bright, clever, feisty and stubborn little girl, but loving and kind to all her friends. At the same time I feel sadness at the frustration I felt during her early weeks. I still experience the sense of powerlessness as I consider the enforced contact of the child development team. I remember how individual practitioners sought to support me, but I felt so disempowered at the lack of faith in their minds about my abilities.

---

1 In the UK, children's centres are a universal service offered to children under five years old and their families, to support their early development.

This story can be viewed as either a reflection of best practice or a reflection of how professionals might manage perceived risk. This experience raises some questions for me:

▶ How can professionals manage service users' feelings of disempowerment and frustration when they receive health services unwillingly?

▶ Do professionals understand the gaps between their perceptions and service users' perceptions of the provision of support?

▶ Do professionals still presume failure among parents with mental ill health?

Providing support to parents with mental health demands a diversity of skilled and knowledgeable responses from health professionals working within multidisciplinary teams. It may comprise professionals from a variety of backgrounds including mental health, maternity and health visiting services, however it's important to remember that some professionals may be less accustomed to working with parents with mental ill health (Darlington *et al*, 2005).

Professionals must respect the mother but prioritise protecting the child (DfE, 2010; 2011). This approach may demand conflicting duties and roles, and indeed mental health professionals often relate more closely to the experiences of parents with mental ill-health while child care professionals can find themselves influenced by more negative stereotypes (Stallard *et al*, 2004), which lead them to fear the parent's potential to abuse or neglect their children (Falkov, 1996).

In my case, child care professionals were managing their fear of working with somebody with schizophrenia, and I felt that they expected me to fail and therefore focused on deficits rather than working from a strengths perspective that assumes success (Fukai *et al*, 2012).

Conclusion

How could practice have been different? I was well, articulate, educated and a registered social worker myself. I was never difficult, angry or oppositional, but I was able to express the powerlessness I felt. Professionals need to have more conversations with service users that both allow them to express their frustration and allow professionals to acknowledge and respond to it. This might build better partnership-working as professionals relate to people who use health services unwillingly.

There could have been more information about the meeting, with greater transparency about the requirements they felt they needed to put in place. The health professionals modified their practice to ensure that I was visited at home by professionals who worked directly with me and also encouraged me to engage with the children's centre. This was a model of good practice but still allowed health professionals to monitor mine and my baby's well-being. However, if professionals had adopted a more hopeful presumption that I could succeed by working from a strengths approach (Fukai *et al*, 2012), rather than presuming the possibility of failure, this would have increased my confidence and addressed some of the powerlessness I felt.

References

Anthony W (1993) Recovery from mental illness: the guiding vision of the mental health service system in the 1990s. *Psychosocial Rehabilitation Journal* **16** (4) 11–23.

Brunner E, Falk DM, Jones M, Dey D & Shatapathy C (2013) Olanzapine in pregnancy and breastfeeding: a review of data from global safety surveillance. *BMC Pharmacology and Toxicology* **14** 38.

Darlington Y, Feeney J & Rixon K (2005) Practice challenges at the intersection of child protection and mental health. *Child and Family Social Work* **10** 239–247.

Department for Education (DfE) (2010) *Munro review of child protection: part 1 – a systems analysis.* London: HMSO.

Department for Education (DfE) (2011) *The Munro Review of Child Protection: Final report. A child-centred system.* London: HMSO.

Falkov A (1996) *Fatal Child Abuse and Parental Psychiatric Disorder: Working Together, Part 8 Reports.* Department of Health ACPC Series, no. 1. London: HMSO.

Fox JR (2012) Best practice in maternity and mental health services? A service user's perspective. *Schizophrenia Bulletin* **38** (4) 651–656.

Fukai S, Goscha R & Rapp, C (2012) Strengths model case management fidelity scores and client outcomes. *Psychiatric Services* **63** 708–710

Gentile S (2010) Antipsychotic therapy during early and late pregnancy. A systematic review. *Schizophrenia Bulletin* **36** (3) 518–544.

Stallard P, Norman P, Huline-Dickens S, Salter E & Cribb J (2004) The effects of parental mental illness upon children: a descriptive study of the views of parents and children. *Clinical Child Psychology and Psychiatry* **9** 39–52.

Chapter 5
Using the Family Model in training: a light bulb moment

By Daphne McKenna

Being a parent

As a trainer, I am always striving for the 'light bulb moment' when a key idea suddenly becomes relevant to practice; the point when a worker realises how a concept or technique can be useful to them, or gains an insight into what something really 'feels' like.

One such 'light bulb moment' happened to me during research as part of the 'Think Child, Think Parent, Think Family' project. I was attempting to gain an understanding from of a group of parents with mental health problems about what help they had found to be effective. They shared their experiences freely, listing their difficulties in getting family members to understand what they were going through and in getting professionals to act to help them. They spoke of the stigma they felt at the school gates and the impact of their condition on all aspects of their lives. All of this I knew but didn't really feel. I know the statistics that between one in four and one in five adults will experience a mental illness during their lifetime (SCIE, 2011). I also know that the simple fact of being married confers more health benefits to men than it does to women (Kiecolt-Glaser & Newton, 2001). In my work as a child protection conference chair I was all too well aware that an estimated one-third to two-thirds of children whose parents have mental health problems will experience difficulties themselves (Dearden & Becker, 2004), so it really ought to have resonated so much more strongly with me.

It wasn't until a woman of about my own age, who was trying to convey the complexity of her experience, said 'you don't stop being a parent just because you're ill', that I was able to truly get a sense that it could be me, and not only that, but if it were me, I wasn't about to stop feeling responsible for my children. It was at that moment that I understood that not only would I continue to worry about my children but was very likely to worry even more; worry about the impact of any mental health condition on them, worry about what I couldn't do for them, worry about how they felt and worry about what they would worry about. It was then that I understood exactly why the Family Model of mental health was such a helpful construct.

Family Model of mental health

As any parent of more than one child knows, children are not born a blank slate. They arrive in the world complete with personality and temperament and they are constantly changing, so their needs are constantly changing too – we can all appreciate that the needs of a toddler are different to the needs of a teenager.

Consequently, the parenting task, the things you have to do for your child, changes over time and for some children it is comparatively easy to meet their needs. However, for some children, the fretful child or the hard to settle, it can be difficult to meet their needs. Where children have complex needs the task is even more demanding. These difficulties and demands impact on us as parents and affect our mental heath (we all have mental health – some days it is better than others – but we all have mental health). These impacts, in turn, unsurprisingly affect our ability to carry out the parenting task – and again unsurprisingly, the way we carry out the parenting task affects the way our child responds, so a cycle of interrelated actions and impacts are set up.

Again, it is axiomatic that children don't live in isolation; they live as members of families. Families also don't live in isolation but are connected to others, however peripherally, as members of society. Societal pressures impact on families for both good and ill. We can think of these pressures in terms of 'stressors' and 'protectors'. Stressors are the pressures bearing down on families such as poverty, ill health or socio-economic disadvantage more generally. Protectors are the societal or environmental advantages that support family functioning, for example adequate housing or a decent education. In truth, the factors we could talk about here are, in essence, 'value neutral'. Housing is a value neutral word but poor housing is a stressor and good housing a protector in this context.

What I have just described is a systems model. The various components all have the potential to interact and affect the other components. The Family Model's importance stems from its ability to help us as practitioners conceptualise the way in which a range of diverse factors relate to one another, in this case how family members might be affected by a parent's experience of mental ill health. It very visually and concretely illustrates the need for a holistic assessment of all elements of the family system and it also starkly demonstrates that change in any one part of the system can have knock-on consequences for the other parts of the system. Similarly, blocks or barriers in one part of the system can have negative consequences for other parts of the system.

Using this model in training

So, as a trainer, how do you help practitioners understand the relevance of this model in such a way as to create a light bulb moment? Not every training course is lucky enough to have service user input. Hearing directly from someone just like you about the impacts of mental illness not only on their lives, but the lives of their partner, children, friends and extended family, leaves a lasting impression. Video clips of real people talking about their real lives is also a powerful tool. However, it is possible to go some way to recreate this experience in a more pedagogic way in the training environment.

'Tell me and I will forget, show me and I may remember, involve me and I will understand.' (Chinese proverb)

Multi-agency training

From experience, multi-agency training is much more effective in helping to make the Family Model a useful tool and in deepening practitioners' understanding of the complexity of life for a family with a parent with mental health problems. Getting staff whose primary focus is work with adults into the same room as staff whose primary focus is children brings numerous advantages. Apart from the obvious benefit of putting names to faces and of increasing understanding of what is and is not possible within different roles and organisations, there are other positive outcomes. The proximity of staff from different disciplines and with different focuses, hearing actual case examples and experiences, helps to challenge preconceptions. Briefly trying to understand what it feels like for that young person, who is in effect an expert in their mother's mental health condition, having their opinion overlooked in discussion, sometimes not even having their presence in the room acknowledged, can be both challenging and illuminating.

Learning, for example, that a mother whose parenting you are critical of delays taking medication so that she is alert enough to read her four-year-old a bedtime story every night, helps you to see her in a more rounded way. Child-focused practitioners are able to demonstrate to their adult-focused colleagues that talking to children is not necessarily a specialist skill. Many adults workers are parents themselves, and we have all been children. Similarly, adult-focused practitioners can help increase understanding of the importance of building a more holistic picture of a parent's functioning, seeing them as a person with hopes and aspirations, and not just as a parent.

Specialist knowledge

It would be unreasonable, however, not to acknowledge that different practitioners have different areas of expertise, based on specialist knowledge. For example, children's practitioners are likely to have a more comprehensive understanding of child development, whereas adult mental health workers will have detailed knowledge about mental health conditions. If working with multi-agency groups, it may be possible for participants to work in pairs to supplement one another's knowledge. Even then it might be helpful to provide handout material detailing the key developmental stages of childhood and the main symptoms and treatment options for the most common mental illnesses. Creating an exercise that requires them to extract information from the handout means that not only do they know they have somewhere to refer to, but also makes them read (at least part of) it.

However, I would add a note of caution here about relying too much on diagnostic labels when assessing risk. It is important to explain in training that labels are just that, and they do not convey the complexity of someone's situation. While many might feel the child living with a parent experiencing schizophrenia is at greater risk than the child living with a depressed parent, this of course depends on a range of other factors. It is possible that a parent experiencing schizophrenia has a great deal of insight into their condition, is compliant with medication and well supported by family members, while a depressed parent may be an isolated care leaver who is self-medicating with alcohol. While no training experience can provide participants with everything they need to know for every situation, it is possible to provide them with the tools to apply principles to one setting that they learnt in another.

Using the model in training and practice

The Family Model helps structure workers' thinking and, in the previous examples, the model would lead practitioners to think about not only the social and environmental circumstances of both the adult and the child, but the impacts of each on the other.

Different disciplines have been trained in the use of different conceptual frameworks and to utilise different assessment models, so it can be difficult to get staff from diverse backgrounds to fully comprehend the perspective of the other. The Family Model has applicability to professionals from all walks of life. Everyone can understand that children grow up in families and that adult service users, if not themselves parents, are likely to be or have been members of a family. They will have been, and will continue to be, affected positively and negatively by the experience of family life. These impacts will have been amplified by the family's socio-economic experiences.

Families will also identify with and benefit from an understanding of the Family Model. Parents can be helped to see how, for example, not taking medication impacts on their ability to manage their child's behaviour and consequently how a child's lack of sleep might precipitate tantrums and prompt a parent to manage their frustration by misuse of alcohol, which in turn affects ability to hold down a job and exacerbates financial problems.

The model can also be used in direct work with children to help illustrate how negative cycles of interaction occur and how a small change might challenge that cycle. It can serve as a tangible tool to help explain how they feel in certain situations and what behaviours have prompted this, enabling the family to identify what changes can be made and by whom.

The Family Model, though it owes its genesis to consideration of the impact of parental mental health on families, has applicability in all family work. The adult may have learning difficulties or be experiencing substance misuse problems. They may be living in a situation of domestic violence or possibly perpetrating domestic violence. Each of these elements will affect their ability to carry out the parenting task, which in turn will shape their child, whose adaptation to a particular style of parenting will soothe or exacerbate the parents' responses. These responses will impact on the family's ability to cope with or take advantage of societal factors.

The challenge for trainers is to convey the many and varied uses of and the range of applications of the Family Model to a variety of social care situations within the confines of a one day training course.

References

SCIE (2011) *Think Child, Think Parent, Think Family: A guide to parental mental health and child welfare* [online]. London: SCIE. Available at: http://www.scie.org.uk/publications/guides/guide30/ (accessed August 2015).

Kiecolt-Glaser JK & Newton TL (2001) Marriage and health: his and hers. *Psychological Bulletin* **127** (4) 472–503.

Dearden C & Becker S (2004) *Young Carers in the UK: the 2004 report* [online]. London: Carers UK and The Children's Society. Available at: http://www.lboro.ac.uk/microsites/socialsciences/ycrg/youngCarersDownload/YCReport2004%5B1%5D.pdf (accessed August 2015).

Policy and drivers for change

Chapter 6

Do recent policy and legislative changes in health and social care help develop the Think Family agenda in parental mental health and child welfare?

By Hugh Constant

Introduction

When we look back, the years 2014–2015 will likely be seen as an important period in the history of social care. In the main this will be because of the Care Act (2014). A few months into the life of the act, it would be premature to judge whether it has had a transformative impact. But the Care Act is indisputably large in scope, and attempts to shift social care decisively towards a personalised model, aimed at promoting the desired outcomes and well-being of everyone who uses the social care system.

The magnitude of the Care Act sometimes makes it feel as if it is the only game in town. But 2014 also saw the introduction of the Children and Families Act (2014), which addresses a number of issues such as adoption, fostering and service integration, and, like the Care Act, it has much to say on young carers.

While new legislation will always garner attention, *Closing the Gap: Priorities for essential change in mental health* (DoH, 2014a) was also released, championed at high levels of government, and is attempting to improve support to people with mental illness, and achieve 'parity of esteem' between mental and physical health.

A busy period, then, for social care and for mental health services. And a busy period too for the Social Care Institute for Excellence (SCIE), a charity improving services to adults and children with care and support needs, and currently heavily involved in supporting Care Act implementation. SCIE also has a long history promoting the 'Think Family' agenda in parental mental health and child welfare, dating back to a 2004 Social Exclusion Unit report into the barriers faced by parents with mental ill health (ODPM, 2014). So, after more than a decade urging people to 'Think Family', how do the new laws and policies help? Can they promote joined-up support to families affected by parental mental illness?

The *Think Child, Think Parent, Think Family* guide

SCIE produced its *Think Child, Think Parent, Think Family* guide into parental mental health and child welfare in 2009. The guide and the evidence underpinning it looked at what works well for families, such as intervening early to prevent difficulties escalating, and helping families to understand mental illness. The guide also explored some of the underlying challenges obstructing whole-family working: inter-agency barriers; a lack of training, knowledge and confidence in working across professional boundaries; workload; and high eligibility thresholds (SCIE, 2009).

Think Child, Think Parent, Think Family made recommendations for front-line staff, managers and senior leaders in the statutory and voluntary sectors across adults' and children's services. It explored how joint working can help throughout any care pathway an adult or child may experience, and made suggestions in areas such as training, communications and strategic leadership. It also set out what good, family-focused services would look like: listening to families' concerns; conducting whole family assessments; working co-operatively across health and social care; making good use of preventative and voluntary services; and taking a strengths-based approach.

What we learnt in practice

From September 2009 to September 2011, SCIE worked with five councils in England and the five health and social care trusts in Northern Ireland to try to implement the *Think Child, Think Parent, Think Family* recommendations. Different areas made different degrees of progress, with Northern Ireland, where the project ran for longer (until March 2012) and was supported and funded at a senior policy and commissioner level, perhaps taking the greatest strides. But all of the sites progressed towards a more family-focused way of addressing parental mental health and child welfare. Advances included new multi-agency family strategies, greater engagement with parents and children in shaping services, new assessment forms that took a family perspective, training initiatives and the embedding of posts within other teams – such as putting family support workers in community mental health teams (SCIE, 2012).

Set against this progress, however, were significant barriers to further developments. The work coincided with the sudden contraction in public funding, so, as the project developed, competing priorities for people's time and money grew, and the senior support that some sites enjoyed early on – and which our evaluation showed was the key determinant of success – did sometimes wane somewhat (SCIE, 2012).

Other barriers included incompatible IT systems, which complicated information-sharing and joined-up assessments, and sometimes a lack of awareness about policy and practice on the 'other' side of the adult mental health and child welfare systems. Also, in systems where performance indicators can really shape priorities, there were no measures that gave precedence to whole-family working.

New legislation and policy

So, to what extent, if any, do the Care Act, the Children and Families Act and the new directives in mental health care help address some of these barriers? Taken individually and collectively, do they give us hope that the Think Family approach to parental mental health and child welfare may be strengthened?

Care Act (2014)

Perhaps the most obvious practice development that *Think Child, Think Parent, Think Family* (SCIE, 2009) called for, and which was found wanting in practice, but is now promoted by the Care Act, is whole family assessments. The act recognises how the situation of the person with care and support needs affects the whole family as an entity. It calls upon local authorities to recognise *'the parenting responsibilities of the person as well as the impact of the adult's needs for care and support on the young carer'* (DoH, 2014b), and thus explicitly reflects the Family Model at the theoretical heart of *Think Child, Think Parent, Think Family* (SCIE, 2009), which recognises the interlinked effects of parent on child, and child on parent, when looking at family well-being.

The Care Act is broad in its interpretation of what constitutes a family when thinking about whole family approaches, citing an authority's duty to identify *'anyone who may be part of the person's wider network of care and support'* (DoH, 2014b) when thinking about who might be affected by the person's care and support needs. There is the potential here to shift the thinking of social care, which has arguably become thoroughly individualised as a spin-off of the necessary push for personalisation. It is a chance to remind ourselves that people typically live in families of one shape or another, and to ignore that ignores the reality of the lives of the people the care system supports.

By focusing on the needs of the whole family, the Care Act necessarily shines a light on the needs of young carers. There is a duty on authorities, where an adult with care and support needs is being assessed, and it appears a child is involved in meeting those needs, to:

→ consider the impact on the child of the disabled adult's needs – in particular, the impact on the child's well-being, welfare, education and development

→ identify whether the child is having to perform tasks which are inappropriate.

(DoH, 2014b)

Based on what is learnt, the authority then has a duty to carry out a young carer's assessment, either under the Care Act (2014), or the Children Act (1989). The Care Act stresses the need to focus on the aspirations of young carers as they enter adulthood themselves (DoH, 2014b), and often that will involve looking at the family system as whole. This sits alongside a general strengthening of the rights of carers under the Care Act, with the potential that creates, to promote the general well-being and resilience of families of people with care and support needs, including mental health problems.

Promoting the use of young carers' assessments in adult social care has the potential to strengthen the sense that the whole family can be the business of an adult department. But the young carer's assessment, with the agreement of all involved, can be conducted by children's services, and this points to a couple of other approaches within the Care Act that, if well used, could help bolster family working. One is the flexibility the act embraces. There is a general philosophy that local authorities and people with care and support needs can jointly determine what the best approach is in any situation, rather than keeping one eye on distantly-derived performance indicators, which rarely include family measures. Another is the very explicit duty throughout the act for statutory bodies to co-operate in the interests of people with care and support needs. We have heard this before, of course. But the act represents another chance for adult and children's social care services, or for an NHS trust and local authority social care team, to work jointly to support a family affected by parental mental illness. The encouragement in the Care Act to pool personal budgets flexibly – which can now come from the NHS and children's services, as well as adult social care – points to one area where creative ideas could be tried out.

The legislative clout that the Care Act gives to whole family approaches has its limits. *Think Child, Think Parent, Think Family* calls for a family eligibility threshold (SCIE, 2009), but eligibility under the act remains on an individual basis alone. And local authorities face challenges in shifting away from processes – not least the computerised information systems on which assessments are recorded – which are absolutely wedded to an individual approach, and which will struggle to flex sufficiently to make family assessments an easy option for time-stretched workers. Furthermore, many adult mental health services are located in NHS trusts, which are perhaps less engaged with the Care Act and its possibilities than local authorities.

But the Care Act focuses more explicitly on parenting than the Fair Access to Care Services rules that it supersedes, by making *'carrying out any caring responsibilities the adult has for a child'* (and stressing that this could be a grandchild, or stepchild) one of the ten key activities that go towards determining eligibility. In that alone, it should help tackle the issue we came across as we tried to implement the Think Family guide, whereby adult workers could simply fail to ask if there were children in the person's life. And the Care Act should also tackle another problem: children's services staff steering clear of adult services because they lack confidence about how the adult social care system works (SCIE, 2012). If nothing else, the Care Act simplifies things, and even that could help bridge gaps between children's and adult services.

Children and Families Act (2014)

The Children and Families Act (2014) may not attract quite the attention of the Care Act, but like it, it is a wide-ranging law, covering adoption, care proceedings, special educational needs and even smoking in cars. But of greatest interest here, arguably, is that, in common with the Care Act, the Children and Families Act opens the way to potentially greater support to young carers. It includes extra duties on local authorities to 'take reasonable steps' to identify young carers, perhaps including things like liaising with schools or (young) carers' organisations. This duty to actively seek young carers who may previously have remained hidden is perhaps of particular benefit to families affected by parental mental ill health, where the needs of the adult, and therefore those of the young carer, can be less obvious.

The act goes on to give young carers a right to an assessment on an 'appearance of need', placing the onus on an authority to reach out to young people. This is new. And the act reinforces the importance of assessing the appropriateness of the young carer's role, and taking into account their educational, employment and leisure needs. It stresses too that their needs can be met directly by support to the young carer, and/or by showing that the cared-for person's care package obviates the need for the young carer's caring input.

In an amendment to the Children Act (1989), the Children and Families Act brings in parent carers' needs assessments, where a child appears to be in need due to their own condition or disability. Given what we know of the evidence that a disability in a child can be an exacerbating factor in a parent's mental ill health (SCIE, 2009), this development may also be of use to parents with mental health problems.

Closing the gap

Moving specifically into the area of mental health, *Closing the Gap: Priorities for essential change in mental health* (DoH, 2014b) aims to give timely and effective support to people experiencing mental illness equal importance to support for the physically unwell. It seeks to build upon 2011's *No Health Without Mental Health* (HM Government, 2011) policy, and unlike the Care Act and the Children and Families Act, it is aspirational, not mandatory. But it too has potential to improve support to parents experiencing mental illness.

Closing the Gap contains 25 priorities for action, such as equity of waiting times for physical and mental health problems. Clearly any improvement of mental health support would generally also improve things for parents with mental health problems by default. So, for example, the drive to ensure that inpatient care takes place closer to home, while proving a real challenge at the moment, is vital to the welfare and cohesion of the family, enabling children to visit parents. Indeed, one great example of practice highlighted in our *Think Family* work was the Barnardo's Young Carers jelly baby logo, in which young carers – and they alone – determined whether family rooms in Liverpool's inpatient mental health facilities were actually family-friendly, and if they were, to paint a jelly baby in the room to celebrate the fact. This seems to be a very visual forerunner of the 'Friends and Family Test' included in *Closing the Gap*.

Perhaps the part of *Closing the Gap* that addresses most directly our concern with parental mental health is that which promises to support new mothers and *'minimise the risks and impacts of postnatal depression'* (DoH, 2014a). Citing the high incident of post- and peri-natal depression, the initiative looks to improve the consistency of people's access to specialist support, and sets Health Education England the target of training sufficient specialists so that every birthing unit has specialist postnatal staff by 2017 (DoH, 2014a). In addition, there is a push for more and better trained health visitors, who can help spot people experiencing postnatal depression at the earliest opportunity.

Conclusion

Achieving Better Access to Mental Health Services by 2020 (DoH, 2014c), which sets out how the goals of *Closing the Gap* (DoH, 2014a) and *No Health Without Mental Health* (HM Government, 2011) might be implemented, identifies an additional £40m funding for 2014/15. Of course, any future funding is subject to the priorities of the new government, but we do know that, despite rising demand, mental health trusts have experienced an 8.25% real-terms reduction in funding from 2010-15 (Community Care, 2015). Such financial pressures can only add to the challenges of fulfilling the various – but wholly compatible – visions of the Care Act, Children and Families Act, and *Closing the Gap*. All three share a goal of personalised, integrated and effective care and support for the people with whom they concern themselves. And all three, separately and combined, therefore hold out the hope for a greater family focus for parents with mental health problems and their children.

Tight budgets are not the only obstacle; whole-family working still requires a shift in thinking from an approach to health and social care that – in adult services particularly – is thoroughly focused on the individual, and not sufficiently cognisant at times of the family context in which people live. SCIE's *Think Child, Think Parent, Think Family* guide set out to tackle that, and much of what it recommended – whole-family assessments, a focus on young carers, awareness-raising about common parental mental health problems such as postnatal depression, and strategic and operational co-operation between adult services and children's social care – is within these new laws and initiatives.

So, as I hope we have shown here, both in their general approaches – integration, flexibility, co-operation – and in their specifics – whole-family assessments, a focus on young carers' aspirations, involving families in assessing mental health services, better postnatal support – the Care Act (2014), the Children and Families Act (2014), and *Closing the Gap* (DoH, 2014a) might just come together to make 2014–15 the start of a good period for whole-family working in parental mental health and child welfare.

References

Community Care (2015) *Mental Health Trust Funding Down 8% From 2010 Despite Coalition's Drive for Parity of Esteem* [online]. Available at: http://www.communitycare.co.uk/2015/03/20/mental-health-trust-funding-8-since-2010-despite-coalitions-drive-parity-esteem/ (accessed August 2015).

Department of Health (2014a) *Closing the Gap: Priorities for essential change in mental health* [online]. London: DoH. Available at: https://www.gov.uk/government/uploads/system/uploads/attachment_data/file/281250/Closing_the_gap_V2_-_17_Feb_2014.pdf (accessed August 2015).

Department of Health (2014b) *Care and Support Statutory Guidance Issued under the Care Act 2014* [online]. London: DoH. Available at: https://www.gov.uk/government/uploads/system/uploads/attachment_data/file/315993/Care-Act-Guidance.pdf (accessed August 2015).

Department of Health (2014c) *Achieving Better Access to Mental Health Services by 2020* [online]. London: DoH. Available at: https://www.gov.uk/government/uploads/system/uploads/attachment_data/file/361648/mental-health-access.pdf (accessed August 2015).

HM Government (2011) *No Health Without Mental Health: A cross-government mental health outcomes strategy for people of all ages* [online]. Available at: https://www.gov.uk/government/uploads/system/uploads/attachment_data/file/213761/dh_124058.pdf (accessed August 2015).

ODPM (2014) *Mental Health and Social Exclusion: Social Exclusion Unit report* [online]. London: Office of the Deputy Prime Minister. Available at: http://www.nfao.org/Useful_Websites/MH_Social_Exclusion_report_summary.pdf (accessed August 2015).

SCIE (2009) *Think Child, Think Parent, Think Family: A guide to parental mental health and child welfare* [online]. Available at: http://www.scie.org.uk/publications/guides/guide30/ (accessed August 2015).

SCIE (2012) *Think Child, Think Parent, Think Family: Final evaluation report.* London: SCIE.

Chapter 7

A change in the law doesn't always mean a change in real lives: making whole family approaches a reality

By Dr Moira Fraser

Louise is a young mum with severe depression[1]. She gets some support from her GP and community mental health team in the form of medication and visits from the team. But for James, her partner, there's little support. He manages everything in the house when Louise is unwell, motivates her to eat, take her medication, and to have a shower and get dressed. James is struggling to work and pay the bills, and worries that his temper is getting short. There is also no support for Jessica, Louise's daughter, who gets herself and her younger sister up, breakfasted and ready for school every day, helps with the cooking and cleaning, sometimes misses school and worries that her mum's depression is her fault. Also needing support is Trisha, Louise's mum, who talks Louise through the difficult times when she sometimes self-harms, and who has her granddaughters to stay, sometimes for weeks at a time, when Louise and James are finding things really difficult.

Thousands of families up and down the country find themselves coping with this kind of situation, doing their best to get through the days. If we're serious about enabling people experiencing mental health problems and their families to stay well and support each other, we've got to do better than this.

Carers and the organisations who support them fought long and hard for the new provisions in law to support carers of all ages in England – both the Care Act (2014) and the Children and Families Act (2014). For the first time in law, unpaid carers looking after family members and friends who can't manage without their help, which includes people experiencing mental health problems, are entitled to an assessment of their needs and support on a par with the rights of the people they care for. Local authorities now have a duty to promote their wellbeing, provide information and advice, assess their needs and where their needs are eligible, draw up support plans and provide that support.

The 2011 Census for England and Wales showed that the proportion of the population providing unpaid care had stayed the same since 2001 – around one in 10 of the population. However the level of caring had increased, with the number of carers providing 50 or more hours of care per week increasing disproportionately (White, 2013). The demographic of the caring population had also changed, with increases in caring amongst the very young (an 83% increase in those aged five to seven years old – yes, you read correctly, five to seven years old) and the very old (a 129% increase in those aged eighty-five or over) (Carers Trust, 2013).

With some of these figures in mind it is a relief that children and young people under 18 who provide unpaid care are also now entitled to support. Many of these are caring for adults – parents or sometimes siblings – with mental health problems. Previously this group was entirely unrecognised in law and as funding for state provision for care became more and more squeezed, we were relying on children to fill the gap with less support and fewer rights than adults in the same position.

We need to ensure that those of all ages who are prepared to care receive the support they need to be able to continue to do so, while maintaining their own health and sense of control over their lives. The new rights are therefore very welcome, and equally welcome is the requirement for local authorities and support services to work in a 'whole family' way.

The statutory guidance to the Care Act (2014), which has the force of law, states:

> 'The intention of the whole family approach is for local authorities to take a holistic view of the person's needs, in the context of their wider support network. The approach must consider both how the adult or their support network or the wider community can contribute towards meeting the outcomes they want to achieve (..), and whether or how the adult's needs for care and support impacts on family members or others in their support network.' (HM Government, 2014, Section 6.43)

---

1 This case study has been created from a composite of real life examples and names have been changed.

This is not without precedent. Services for young carers have been promoting whole family approaches for years, recently for example, through the Department for Education funded Making a Step Change programme, run by Carers Trust and The Children's Society (2015). Our policy aim for young carers has been to reduce caring roles which are harmful – either because they mean a child can't get to school or take part in activities like other children, because they feel stigmatised or bullied, or because they become unwell, physically or mentally. There is limited point in supporting a young carer in isolation from the rest of their family. While activities and breaks are welcome, they are only of minimal help if the young person then has to go back to the same difficult situation they have come from, with no prospect of that improving.

Efforts should therefore focus on ensuring that where there is a young carer with needs, support is put in place to help the adults in that environment, thus reducing the caring role of the child. This process is now reinforced in law, and the Care Act (2014) and Children and Families Act (2014) should work in tandem to put this in place for all young carers and their families.

However, whole family approaches are not just about children and young people. We can see from other approaches elsewhere – such as circles of support (Burke, 2006) – that it is relevant wherever a person of any age has needs and is being supported by a range of family and friends in a range of ways. Almost all of us, except for the most isolated, live in interdependent relationships based on mutual support, acting and interacting in different ways at different times. Focusing on only one person in that dynamic was always a strange concept. In all likelihood, underneath this lies a deficit model related to an individual's condition. Fix the deficit, or plug the gap caused by the deficit, and the job's seen to be done, But beyond this gap identified by services, is often an unacknowledged and vast range of support – macro and micro – which people do for themselves, or which family, friends and neighbours do. This support makes it possible for a person to manage all the other aspects of their lives and stay as well and independent as they can, and it only takes one of those supporting bricks to wobble, and it can be the start of complete collapse.

So, let's go back to the family we started with – Louise, James, their two daughters and Louise's mum, Trisha. Support for Louise is vital, of course, but James, Jessica and Trisha are people with needs too. They all play their crucial part in making their family work, and they all deserve support in a way which joins up in the same way their family does; without artificial boundaries and barriers.

The legislation is now in place to provide that support. However, my concern is that legislation on its own is does not effect change – people do. Many pieces of legislation have made it as far as the statute book but made little difference to people's lives. The aim therefore has to be that at least some of the positive intentions of the law turn into practical action which transforms lives.

What we have to tackle is multiple systemic and cultural barriers. Social care and health services were essentially designed for individual practitioners to meet individuals' needs. In some areas we are getting closer to teams working collaboratively with individuals – such in as in multidisciplinary community mental health teams, where they are effectively resourced and led. In children's areas, we are getting better at working in whole teams with whole families, at least in terms of the rhetoric, but in other areas we are still as far off as ever.

A key way forward in supporting young carers has been the introduction the Memorandum of Understanding (ADCS, ADASS, the Children's Society and Carers Trust, 2015) – where local authority children's and adult services agree ways of working together to support families – which often has been more difficult than it sounds to achieve. The Care Act now requires adult social workers to do the previously unthinkable and to actively recognise children – young carers – in the course of working with adults with care needs. I don't underestimate the cultural challenge and there is a risk that hard-pressed social workers may be left feeling under-supported and overwhelmed.

Still we face challenges within social care services or within NHS services for people of all ages, where services meet the administrative needs of the service, but not those of the person and family in whose interests the services are supposedly provided. We still have systems which seem incapable of talking to each other, leaving families to do the patching together. This creates even more stress and frustration, where the point of provision of services was to reduce this. The integration agenda, where health and social care should be more joined up to improve outcomes, has to be the right way forward and perhaps new moves such as local devolution (where health and care economies can work through local solutions) may offer the best hope of success.

Of course, in all of this we can't ignore the crisis in social care funding. With less and less to go round, it is hard to ask social workers or others to do more even if it would improve outcomes. Most people care desperately about their work and so keep trying, but we have a system on the brink of collapse. Successive governments have failed to tackle it properly because the solutions are politically unpalatable. Social care is not a subject people want to talk about – it's about things which are private, embarrassing and happen in the privacy of our own homes. So the issue remains low on the political agenda but unless we address it, demands on social care, the NHS, community services and families will increase. So, I fear, will instances of the most isolated members of our communities struggling or failing to cope in the direst of circumstances.

In all of this we must try to take some positives. Whole family approaches, with the force of law given by the Care Act and its guidance, offer a torch of hope that an underpinning principle has been established and can be built on, culturally and practically. With more and more care being provided by families – James, Jessica, Trisha and the many thousands like them – along with the other issues families face in a climate where the support services they once relied on and trusted are disappearing, we need all the positives we can hang onto.

References

ADCS, ADASS, The Children's Society & Carers Trust (2015) *No Wrong Doors; Working together to support young carers and their families* [online]. Available at: http://www.local.gov.uk/documents/10180/11431/No+wrong+doors+-+working+together+to+support+young+carers+and+their+families/d210a4a6-b352-4776-b858-f3adf06e4b66 (accessed September 2015).

Burke C (2006) *Building Community through Circles of Friends: A practical guide to making inclusion a reality for people with learning disabilities* [online]. London: Foundation for People with Learning Disabilities. Available at: http://mentalhealth.org.uk/content/assets/PDF/publications/building-community.pdf?view=Standard (accessed September 2015).

Carers Trust (2013) *Census 2011: Provision of unpaid care, Carers Trust briefing* [online]. Available at: http://www.adass.org.uk/AdassMedia/stories/Carers/Census%202011%20briefing%20Age%20statistics%2016%2005%202013.pdf (accessed September 2015).

Carers Trust and the Children's Society (2015) *Making a Step Change: Putting it into practice* [online]. Available at: http://makingastepchange.info/ (accessed September 2015).

HM Government (2014) *The Care Act* [online]. Available at: www.legislation.gov.uk/ukpga/2014/23/contents/enacted/data.htm (accessed October 2015)

White C (2013) 2011 *Census Analysis: Unpaid care in England and Wales, 2011 and comparison with 2001* [online]. Office for National Statistics. Available at: http://www.ons.gov.uk/ons/dcp171766_300039.pdf (accessed September 2015).

Chapter 8

What has happened to 'Think Family': challenges and achievements in implementing family inclusive practice

By Dr Jerry Tew, Professor Kate Morris, Professor Sue White, Professor Brid Featherstone and Sarah-Jane Fenton

In 2008, the Cabinet Office published *Think Family: A literature review of whole family approaches* (Morris *et al*, 2008), which informed further analysis and policy papers that sought to encourage a more holistic and contextualised understanding of people's lives, and more joined-up approaches to delivering services – especially for those families who were experiencing multiple challenges (Cabinet Office, 2007; 2008). Underpinning this was a set of key principles:

→ A broad and flexible understanding of 'family' as a relational network of significant others who may or may not have ties of kinship or marriage, and may or may not be co-resident.

→ A recognition that all family members need to be seen as people in their own right with multiple roles and relationships inside and outside the family.

→ A focus on *'relationships between different family members [that] uses family strengths to limit negative impacts of family problems and encourages progress towards positive outcomes'* (Cabinet Office, 2007, p30).

→ 'No wrong door' – a 'whole family' assessment of need and capabilities irrespective of referral route(s).

This was in stark contrast to the explicit and implicit direction of most other government policy and guidance, which had increasingly individualised the ways in which need and risk were understood – and hence how services were supposed to be delivered in response to these (see, for example, Morris, 2011). Policy and service responses in relation to families had been becoming increasingly institutionally fragmented, with responsibility split between government departments (health, education, justice, work and pensions, communities and local government) that were then reproduced at local level, with practice being driven by a confusing and disconnected matrix of separate targets, funding streams and service thresholds.

Prevailing discourses tended to focus on the paramount importance of the child ('every child matters' not 'every family matters'), or on the vulnerable adult (whose profile of need and risk was to be assessed on an individual rather than a relational basis). Responsibility (and blame) for matters such as risk and anti-social behaviour could be located with specific individuals – often with a single identified parent or carer (who could often be powerless and over-stretched) – rather than with wider relational systems that might have had greater capacity to address and resolve complex and inter-related issues were they given appropriate support and opportunities.

The analysis identified a range of approaches to 'family' within services that could be characterised as an ascending 'ladder' of family inclusiveness:

1. A predominant focus on an identified individual with other family members being consulted and expected to provide support.

2. A focus on the separate needs of different family members (e.g. individual assessments for service user and identified 'carer') and/or on specific 'axial relationships' (Cornford *et al*, 2013) – i.e. dyads such as parent-child, carer-vulnerable adult, in which one party can tend to be seen mainly in relation to their designated role (as carer or parent).

3. Engagement with family as a relational network of significant others.

(Cabinet Office, 2007, p30)

Within the literature review (Morris *et al*, 2008), it was recognised that many service models and policy initiatives with 'family' in their titles had tended to fall within levels 1 and 2 – with an increasing focus on parents and informal carers (and on the activities of caring and parenting), but with relatively few examples that created the space in which to explore the wider relational contexts of people's family lives.

What has happened since 'Think Family': taking stock

The Family Potential Research Centre recently obtained funding from the Economic and Social Research Council (ESRC) for a programme of knowledge exchange activity around the theme of family inclusive policy and practice (see www.familypotential.org). Our first seminar provided an opportunity, with a broad range of stakeholders, to take stock of developments and challenges since the launch of the Think Family policy initiative in 2008. These developments have involved an interesting combination of 'headline' initiatives at a policy level, together with 'bottom-up' activity at a local level where people have sought to take forward new and more inclusive ways of working.

The headline developments initially included Family Pathfinder projects (based on the earlier Family Intervention Project model that targeted families with multiple and complex needs who were also seen as disruptive to the wider community) and the *Think Child, Think Parent, Think Family* pilots (that sought to integrate family support where both children's and mental health services were potentially involved) (see SCIE, 2012). Although an inclusive 'whole family focus' initially lost prominence at the start of the coalition government, family-focused thinking resurfaced in the form of the Troubled Families initiative that built on the Family Intervention Project model, but introduced education and employment as an explicit additional focus. Perceived as a success (although we await the final evaluation report), the government has now rolled out phase 2 of the programme with a significantly broadened remit.

Most recently, a very explicit family inclusive focus has been introduced in joint guidance from the Department of Health, the Local Government Association, the Association of Directors of Adult Social Services, the Children's Society and the Carers' Trust on the implementation of the Care Act (2014) using whole-family approaches (DoH *et al*, 2015). While the Care Act, along with the Children and Families Act (2014), provides a framework for the specific consideration of young carers in a whole family context, its ambition is much wider. It states that local authorities are required to *'adopt a whole system, whole council, whole-family approach, co-ordinating services and support around the person'* (DoH *et al*, 2015, p7). Within the Care Act and this guidance, there is a determined attempt to introduce a positive and preventative focus on building resilience and well-being, rather than a deficit focus on need and risk.

Beneath the headlines, we have seen a number of other developments, sometimes swimming with the tide, using headline policies to their advantage but often also having to struggle against the impact of other policies, such as austerity, both on families and mainstream support services.

These developments have included Family Recovery Projects that have sought to frame the intensive family support message in a rather more positive way – with an explicit focus on family assets and potential, while also recognising families' troubles. Unlike earlier Family Intervention Projects, where unresolved mental health issues had often emerged as a sticking point (Lloyd *et al*, 2011), this approach has included mental health and substance misuse expertise within the core team (Thoburn *et al*, 2011).

Similar thinking and practice has also emerged, in some areas, within local approaches to the Troubled Families Initiative (Tew, 2013), and has also featured in some of the Big Lottery-funded 'Improving Futures' locality-based projects that have sought to mobilise the resources of the voluntary sector around families in their communities (Hughes, 2015).

Although geographically patchy, there has been substantial expansion of Family Group Conferencing activity with support from both local authorities and organisations such as the Family Rights Group. This offers a democratic and inclusive process for family decision making and the model has now been developed for use in making decisions relating to the care of vulnerable adults and supporting the recovery of people with mental distress (Barnsdale & Walker, 2007; Morris & Connolly, 2010; De Jong & Schout, 2011). A more recent development – so far just taking off within mental health services – is the 'Open Dialogue' approach, which originates from Finland and in which the focus for all support, intervention and decision making is a series of ongoing (and initially frequent) meetings with the person and their relational network (Seikkula *et al*, 2006). Although emerging from very different cultural origins (the New Zealand Maori and Western Lapland communities respectively), there are some very interesting commonalities within the values and practices that characterise these two approaches, including a commitment to include all significant others and not just immediate family, and a willingness to share power and ensure that all voices are heard and taken into account.

However, the continuation of a risk-averse climate within local authority children's services, combined with a policy focus on the primary need to protect children from the harms posed by their parents' actions or inactions, has meant that family-focused approaches are struggling to be developed more widely in this sector. The focus on the protection needs of children, as distinct from the support needs of their family, has been exacerbated by the impact on practice of information and computer systems in use in local authorities and by particular organisational approaches to accountability (Broadhurst *et al* 2010; Hall *et al*, 2010; White *et al*, 2010).

Protecting children, and increasingly rescuing them from their failing parents, has been an explicit theme in government policy in England in recent years (Featherstone *et al*, 2014). This has been reflected in a shift in resources in a harsh spending climate towards adoption, with investment in birth families appearing to be less of a priority – although the UK has been criticised by the Council for Europe for its use of non-consensual adoption in cases of maternal mental illness and domestic abuse (Council for Europe, 2015). This prioritising of adoption over family support has been legitimated through the rising influence of neuro-biological rather than socio-political explanatory frameworks (Wastell & White, 2012) with a surprising degree of support from across much of the political spectrum. The following quotation from social democratic Scotland gives a flavour of the prevailing moral context:

'... we now know that there is a strong link between antenatal anxiety and maternal depression, and poor outcomes for children including development, parental bonding and behavioural problems.'
(Scottish Government, 2015)

Despite these countervailing tendencies, there have also been positive moves towards whole-family working through, for example, the engagement with restorative approaches in some local authorities. Such approaches are rooted in an understanding of, and a commitment to, fostering the relational connections of individuals and to supporting families to care safely and flourish (Wardell, 2015). Alongside this, systemic approaches to working with families have become embedded in a range of local authorities as a result of rolling out the 'Reclaim Social Work' model, which promotes systemic family therapy as a key method of practice (Goodman & Trowler, 2011).

Challenges and achievements in taking forward the Think Family agenda

The seminar provided a forum for a cross-section of practitioners, managers and other stakeholders to flag up their particular experiences of what had been achieved and the challenges that they faced. Out of this, a number of common themes emerged, both in relation to thinking holistically about family networks and around the practicalities of implementing more family-inclusive approaches in terms of policies and practices.

A number of delegates shared their experiences of striving to widen the idea of 'family' beyond a narrow focus on parents (usually mothers) and parenting, or singular 'carers' and vulnerable adults. However, this was not always easy within a wider context in which expectations around evidence-based practice tended to promote a degree of tunnel-vision, with pressure to focus on discrete interventions that had been experimentally validated, such as parenting programmes, but which only engaged with a small part of the complexity of families' lives. Alongside this was the need to continually rethink family in the context of different communities, cultures and demographics – and to understand the reality of 'doing family' from the perspective of the lived experience of vulnerable families facing multiple challenges (Morris, 2012).

Arguing for broader whole-family thinking could be difficult because of a lack of 'acceptable' evidence on the effectiveness of messy, flexible, joined-up, relationship-based, whole systems practice. The lack of standardisation inherent in responding to the unique assets and challenges of a particular family situation makes it somewhat problematic to construct an evaluation using a medical-style randomised controlled trial (RCT) methodology. Nevertheless, evidence at a whole service/whole community level suggests that a genuinely inclusive and relational mode of practice can produce quite dramatically high success rates, as in the case of the Open Dialogue service in Finland where recovery rates from serious mental illness are between two and three times higher than the European norm (Seikkula et al, 2006).

A major challenge was seen to be shifting the focus of organisational culture from streamlining services into standardised and narrowly focused interventions ('production line' model), to one that promotes and enables holistic solution-focused engagement with families. Within some organisations, middle management could inadvertently become a 'roadblock to change' – having only been trained to manage a fragmented 'production line' service and how to enforce a procedural practice that focuses on individual needs or risks, and the achievement of targets.

Despite changes in government (and rhetoric), there has nevertheless been real continuity in developing positive, asset-based/strengths-based thinking and practice – and many delegates were able to share the achievements of locally based projects and services. Relational network focused models, such as Family Group Conferencing, systemic practice, Team around the Family, and Open Dialogue, have been gaining traction in many localities, and practitioners are getting more confident and capable in family-focused approaches. They are deriving pride from being able to give families time and space to resolve their difficulties, and are seeing this making a difference in terms of helping to bring about positive and sustainable outcomes. However, this raises the challenge of how to embed and sustain such family inclusive ways of working within local service systems, and also to find a new language for (joint) commissioning as families do not fit into 'care pathways', diagnostically related groups, or narrow individualised notions of risk and need. Alongside this there is a need to find workable solutions to issues of service thresholds and criteria for eligibility, so that families facing multiple and complex challenges do not just fall through the net.

The impact of austerity was seen by participants as double edged. On the one hand, loss of funding threatens many of the more informal voluntary sector support services that have enabled families to carry on functioning in the community. Although facing their own cuts, mainstream but more individually focused services, such as health and child protection, can remain relatively protected in terms of ongoing core funding, whereas innovative projects engaging with whole families – however successful – may be reliant on time-limited funding (e.g. from the Big Lottery). On the other hand, the very scale of the funding crisis means that the downwards 'salami slicing' of existing service provision may look increasingly unfeasible, and more innovative statutory authorities (such as West Berkshire) may seize this as an opportunity to re-conceive ways of delivering services: looking for creative and co-productive solutions by engaging very differently with families and communities (Wardell, 2015). If the transaction at the 'front door' emphasises families' potential for agency and capability, it can be much easier to engage with families in ways that are co-productive and less stigmatising. However, if you get the 'front door' wrong, it may take a lot of work to undo the damage done.

Perhaps the most unexpected thing to emerge from the seminar was the level of unhelpful opposition, particularly (but not exclusively) from within the field of children and family services, and the conflict between those undertaking family support and social work roles – with social work intervention being construed as a threat (by both family support workers and social workers themselves), to be brought in if families did not make sufficient progress on their own account. This may come out in a jostling for status and recognition – or 'practitioner envy' – but may reflect a deeper conflict of values and orientations in which, somewhat bizarrely, social workers may be inducted into the role of being the custodians of an individualising focus on child or adult protection, and using their status within organisations to 'pull rank' over those seeking to enable families to find collective and sustainable solutions to their difficulties. This highlights three things: a lack of skills and (joint) training to support relationship-based ways of working; a need to challenge the notion that, in some way, 'family support' is not as skilled as 'family intervention'; and the importance of seeing family support as integral to the role of social work (see Featherstone et al, 2013).

Looking forward

The roll-out of the second phase of the Troubled Families programme and the guidance on *The Care Act and Whole-Family Approaches* (DoH et al, 2015) both provide valuable levers for whole system change in how local authorities engage with families – potentially bridging organisational splits between health, social care and criminal justice systems, and between children's and adults' services. However, implementing new ways of thinking about and responding to families may raise huge challenges for local authorities and other agencies that are steeped in more individualised and fragmented ways of working. Some may seek to 'do the minimum' rather than venture into somewhat uncharted territory. Some may choose to move forward but in more limited ways, concentrating just on (a) those families that meet the criteria for implementing the next phase of the Troubled Families programme and (b) the implementation of joined-up, whole-family support services around young carers in compliance with the requirements of the Care Act and the Children and Families Act.

There is an urgent need to research and learn from the experience of those localities that are at the forefront of implementing new approaches and ways of working – and particularly where a whole-family approach comes to be seen as first response rather than a last resort. It is to be hoped that this will lead to a greater shared ownership of the Think Family agenda across services and a rebalancing of the assumption that it is only families with children that matter. In turn, these developments may serve to shine more of a spotlight on the current disjunction in approach between much of family support and child protection activity – including moving beyond the limitations of the Children's Assessment Framework (CAF) and current organisational and ICT systems within child protection that can militate against taking an effective systemic or whole-family perspective. At a more fundamental level, it may encourage a shift from a potentially punitive way of working to one that is more embedded within the principles of restorative practice.

In order to take the agenda forward, there is a need to refine our conceptual understanding – including how to maintain a 'level 3' whole-family approach rather than conflating this with a 'level 2' focus on specific family members and their axial relationships (as may be the case with, say, parenting programmes). In moving beyond a reactive, deficit-based approach, it may be important to develop a coherent (and operationally useful) understanding of primary, secondary and tertiary prevention across the life course, rather than an over-emphasis on early years intervention and a consequent neglect of what may be achieved subsequently – particularly around points of transition within families' life-cycles. Speaking of similar developments in the US, which predate those in the UK by some decades, Bruer argues: *'Overemphasizing the importance of the first three years … amounts to thinking about and attacking problems from an artificially limited perspective and a limited armamentarium of possible interventions'* (Bruer, 1999, pp.173–4). A focus on the first three years can create 'cliff edges' of intervention and squeeze out resources from helping whole families across the life course (Wastell & White, 2012)

Equally pressing is the need both to make best use of the existing evidence base and to identify the gaps within this – and for practitioners, advocacy organisations and families themselves to have a voice in formulating the research questions that would actually make a difference in enabling families to prosper more effectively. For many practitioners and managers, the key concern is how to assess effectiveness and cost-effectiveness – in order to make the case for family inclusive approaches and to identify what works best within these. There may be a need for a paradigm shift in terms of developing more sophisticated evaluation methodologies that can capture the complexity of relational/whole-systems work and which shift the agenda beyond a reductionist 'drug trial' RCT type model (with a single 'primary outcome' measure) and which look at a more comprehensive evaluation of process and potentially multiple outcomes, perhaps including a 'Theories of Change' analysis of the 'steps along the way' that may be necessary in order to achieve such outcomes.

Finally, there needs to be recognition of a considerable training and skills agenda. Whether one is a systemically oriented social worker, a family group conference facilitator, an open dialogue practitioner or a community-based family support worker, one has to learn how to feel comfortable being with whole, extended and/or fragmented families – groups of people with complex histories and inter-relationships and with potentially conflicting needs, agendas and aspirations. This is a pre-requisite for being able to do anything constructive in terms of engaging with families as relational networks – and can often be missing from the professional training of social workers and other practitioners. Indeed, learning to be with a family group or network may involve unlearning significant elements of professional training or customary practice. Without addressing this agenda, it may prove surprisingly hard to translate family inclusive policy initiatives into consistent and effective practice on the ground.

References

Barnsdale L & Walker M (2007) *Examining the Use and Impact of Family Group Conferencing*. Edinburgh: Scottish Executive.

Bruer JT (1999) *The Myth of the First Three Years*. The Free Press, New York.

Broadhurst K, Wastell D, White S, Hall C, Peckover S, Thompson K, Pithouse A & Davey D (2010) Performing 'initial assessment': identifying the latent conditions for error at the front-door of local authority children's services. *British Journal of Social Work* **40** (2) 352–370.

Cabinet Office (2007) *Reaching Out: Think family. Analysis and themes from the Families at Risk review*. London: Cabinet Office Social Exclusion Task Force.

Cabinet Office (2008) *Think Family: Improving the life chances of families at risk.* London: Cabinet Office Social Exclusion Task Force.

Cornford J, Baines S & Wilson R (2013) Representing the family: how does the state 'think family'? *Policy & Politics* **41** (1) 1–18.

Council for Europe (2015) *Social Services in Europe: Legislation and practice of the removal of children from their families in Council of Europe member States* [online]. Available at: http://website-pace.net/documents/10643/1127812/EDOC_Social+services+in+Europe.pdf/dc06054e-2051-49f5-bfbd-31c9c0144a32 (accessed September 2015).

De Jong G & Schout G (2011) Family group conferences in public mental health care: An exploration of opportunities. *International Journal of Mental Health Nursing* **20** (1) 63–74.

Department of Health, Local Government Association, ADASS, the Children's Society & Carers' Trust (2015) *The Care Act and Whole-Family Approaches* [online]. Available at: http://www.local.gov.uk/documents/10180/5756320/The+Care+Act+and+whole+family+approaches/080c323f-e653-4cea-832a-90947c9dc00c (accessed September 2015).

Featherstone B, Morris K & White S (2013) A Marriage Made in Hell: early intervention meets child protection. *British Journal of Social Work* doi: 10.1093/bjsw/bct052.

Featherstone B, White S & Morris K (2014) *Re-imagining Child Protection: Towards humane social work with families.* Bristol: Policy Press.

Goodman S & Trowler I (2011) *Social Work Reclaimed: Innovative frameworks for child and family social work practice.* London: Jessica Kingsley.

Hall C, Parton N, Peckover S & White S (2010) Child-centric ICTs and the fragmentation of child welfare practice in England. *Journal of Social Policy* **39** (3) 393–413.

Hughes S (2015) *Big Manchester: Developing family minded practices* [online]. University of Birmingham: Family Potential Research Centre. Available at: http://www.familypotential.org/?page_id=29 (accessed September 2015).

Lloyd C, Wollny I, White C, Gowland S & Purdon S (2011) *Monitoring and Evaluation of Family Intervention Services and Projects Between February 2007 and March 2011* [online]. London: Department for Education. Available at: https://www.gov.uk/government/uploads/system/uploads/attachment_data/file/184031/DFE-RR174.pdf (accessed September 2015).

Morris K (2011) Thinking Family? The complexities of family engagement in care and protection. *British Journal of Social Work.* 10.1093/bjsw/bcr116.

Morris K (2012) Troubled families: vulnerable families' experiences of multiple service use. *Child and Family Social Work.* doi: 10.1111/j.1365-2206.2011.00822.

Morris K & Connolly M (2010) Family decision-making in child welfare: challenges in developing a knowledge-base for practice. *Child Abuse Review* DOI: 10.1002/car.1143.

Morris K, Hughes N, Clarke H, Tew J, Mason P, Galvani S, Lewis A & Loveless L (2008) *Think Family: A literature review of whole family approaches.* Cabinet Office Social Exclusion Task Force.

Scottish Government (2015) *Consultation on the draft Statutory Guidance for Parts 4, 5 and 18 (Section 96) and related draft orders of the Children and Young People (Scotland) Act 2014* [online]. Available at: http://www.gov.scot/Publications/2015/02/1851/14 (accessed September 2015).

SCIE (2012) *Think Child, Think Parent, Think Family: Final evaluation report* [online]. London: SCIE. Available at: http://www.scie.org.uk/publications/reports/report56.pdf (accessed September 2015).

Seikkula J, Aaltonen J, Alakare B, Haarakangas K, Keränen J & Lehtinen K (2006) Five-year experience of first-episode non-affective psychosis in open-dialogue approach: treatment principles, follow-up outcomes, and two case studies. *Psychotherapy Research* **16** (2) 214–228.

Tew J (2013) Asset based approaches and 'troubled families': can the discourses join up? *Families, Relationships and Societies* **2** (3) 467–470.

Thoburn J, Cooper N, Connolly S & Brandon M (2011) *Process and Outcome Research on the Westminster Family Recovery Pathfinder* [online]. Norwich: University of East Anglia. Available at: http://democracy.lbhf.gov.uk/documents/s22804/Item%2012f%20-%20BP%20Report%20final%20Nov%202011.pdf (accessed September 2015).

Wardell R (2015) *Perspectives from the Field* [online]. University of Birmingham: Family Potential Research Centre. Available at: http://www.familypotential.org/?page_id=29 (accessed September 2015).

Wastell D & White S (2012) Blinded by neuroscience: social policy and the myth of the infant brain. *Families, Relationships and Societies* **1** (3) 397–414.

White S, Wastell D, Broadhurst K & Hall C (2010) When policy o'erleaps itself: the 'tragic tale' of the integrated children's system. *Critical Social Policy* **30** (3) 405–429.

Children and early intervention

Chapter 9

Children should be seen and heard in adult mental health services

By Ragni Whitlock and Dr Estelle Rapsey

Introduction

There is growing recognition of children's needs where a parent has mental health difficulties. Beardslee et al (1998) conducted a ten-year literature review looking at the effects of parental affective illness on children and concluded that these children are at a greater risk of psychiatric disorders than the children of non-ill parents. Indeed, children who are aware of their parent's mental health difficulties can often feel confused, scared, angry and powerless to change the situation (The Children's Society Survey, 2008). There are several government publications such as *Think Child, Think Parent, Think Family* (SCIE, 2011), and helpful resources and programmes offered by charitable organisations such as Barnado's, yet the routine identification and inclusion of children in our adult mental health services remains scant.

The historical and working context

We, the authors of this paper, Ragni and Estelle, are clinical staff members employed in adult mental health (AMH) services in Somerset Partnership Trust. Estelle is a clinical psychologist and Ragni a family therapist. Both of us have a passion for systemic work, an approach that favours the inclusion of the patient's family and social network, both for understanding the relational aspects of well-being and for working towards recovery. We work in the rural county of Somerset, which nestles beneath the rolling Mendip, Blackdown and Quantock hills, and has a population of about 520,000.

Our service offers a range of established systemic interventions. Family therapy clinics were first set up in the 1980s to cover the four rural localities: Taunton, Somerset Coast, South Somerset and Mendip. Later developments included an integrated family interventions service for psychosis (see Burbach & Stanbridge, 1998; 2006) and a carers' support service. In 2002, a trust strategy to enhance working partnerships with families and carers' was agreed, prompting the development of an inpatient staff training programme on family and carer awareness for all adult mental health wards. While this resulted in initial changes in staff confidence and raised awareness about the need to include families in routine practice, it remained a challenge to influence the ward culture away from a patient-centric view towards a family and carer inclusive view. To address this, 'specialist' family liaison workers were introduced to work alongside and train inpatient staff. This offered families and carers a meeting at which they could talk about their needs and to give and receive information about the patient (Stanbridge, 2012). At this point, the importance of collecting information about any children who are in regular contact with a patient was recognised, and has since become routine practice. Having information about the presence of children was a first step to recognising the needs of children who were carers and enabled signposting to child-focused services such as young carers support groups.

We are continuing to develop our 'Family Liaison' model by extending it into the community teams. We also offer 'Family Liaison Plus', where up to three systemic meetings may be offered (brief, low-intensity systemic work) if the initial family liaison meeting has brought issues to the fore that need some brief therapeutic intervention. This has been accomplished by having a small team of systemic specialists available to join with or consult to front-line staff in holding systemic meetings for couples and families.

These brief systemic interventions help to establish the 'Triangle of Care' (Worthington *et al*, 2013) between staff, patient and family, and also help to share information, open up channels of communication and begin to explore patterns of relating and communicating that may have become unhelpful.

Family Liaison sessions can be offered as stand-alone meetings or can lead to formal referrals to the family therapy clinics if longer term, formalised systemic work is indicated. This will usually be for patients and families who are presenting with more complex needs or greater relational difficulties. This enables us to offer family inclusive practice on a continuum basis, utilising a 'stepped care' model where clients and their support networks can access lower or higher intensities of systemic work, therefore 'stepping up' to services depending on the presenting difficulties and complexities (Burbach, 2015).

Many of the developments in Somerset predate national policies e.g. *Think Family* (Cabinet Office, 2008) yet it seems that routinely identifying children in adult mental health services remains limited. This is in comparison to government initiatives such as *What About the Children* (Ofsted, 2013) where it is mandatory in adult services to collect information about children where there is a drug or alcohol problem.

Children below the radar

Locally, both our inpatient wards and community teams now endeavour to ask families and patients about children, however children have seldom been directly included in family meetings. This exclusion seems to reflect the past ethos of adult mental health services generally. In our view, the individual-oriented culture of adult services in which a single adult is the identified patient has led to a focus on individual therapies within adult services, and a diminishment or even disappearance of the patient's social network, particularly the children connected with the adult's life, who are usually part of the patient's own family. Although initiatives and various governmental policies have brought about the greater inclusion of families and carers, it still remains that the majority of identified carers within our mental health services are adults. Through our own therapeutic work with family systems we have become aware of the children who fall below the radar or who do not reach the threshold for their own services or support.

We have been keen to remedy this situation. We have become increasingly interested in thinking about and finding ways to include children within the systemic work delivered for adult mental health, and within that work to be oriented to the well-being of the whole social network – adults and children, patients, partners and offspring. In addition, Ragni's previous CAMHS experience has promoted a growing awareness that, where appropriate, it is both useful and important to include the children in the meetings we hold, not only because their needs may easily be overlooked but also because they are often a key element of a patient's social system. Thus, there is growing focus on the needs of these children within our services and greater effort to include them more actively in our thinking and in our systemic approaches.

The systemic approach

Underpinning a systemic approach is an assumption about the reciprocity of relationships: the idea that, within families or social systems, behaviour and relationships are contingent upon each other in a circular way. Through a systemic lens the well-being of the child and the well-being of the adult in a family are connected; each affects and is affected by the other (figure 1).

Thus, when the mental health of a parent declines we may see an increase of physical health symptoms in a child such as tummy aches, or an increase of behavioural problems or the deterioration of the child's own mental health. This in turn will affect the well-being and recovery of the adult patient.

The following vignettes outline what we believe to be some of the key aims of including children in systemic work for adult mental health. These vignettes are taken from our direct experience of working systemically with families but are not specific to any one family. This has been done to provide anonymity and conceal identities.

Helping children to understand mental health issues in a child friendly way

In 2006, Somerset Partnership joined forces with the local Young Carers Project to develop 'Listen to ME!' rucksacks for children and young people visiting family in our inpatient wards. These contained age-appropriate workbooks and information on mental health difficulties. The hope is that when staff hand these out to young people it will improve the young person's experience and understanding of mental health services and raise staff and carer awareness about the impact of parental mental health difficulties on children. The rucksacks provide accessible information about mental health issues and tools to help staff and family members speak with young people about mental health problems.

Support for the parenting patient and parenting couple in managing parenting tasks alongside mental health difficulties

Sam and his wife, Janette, came to the family therapy clinic (out-patient) with their two sons, Evan (14) and Michael (12). Sam was suffering from chronic anxiety, OCD symptoms and depression. This was having a significant impact on their family life together and in particular Sam's role as a father. The two boys talked about missing the time they used to spend with their Dad before his illness. We discussed with Sam and Janette how they as a couple could work towards Sam having quality time with the boys within the limitations imposed by his illness. For example, how an activity that Sam was still able to enjoy with this eldest son could become more frequent and be expanded to create a sense of shared purpose and enjoyment. In addition, we looked at the way in which spending this time together would improve the relationship between Sam and his son and as well as improving Sam's sense of agency and well-being.

Figure 1

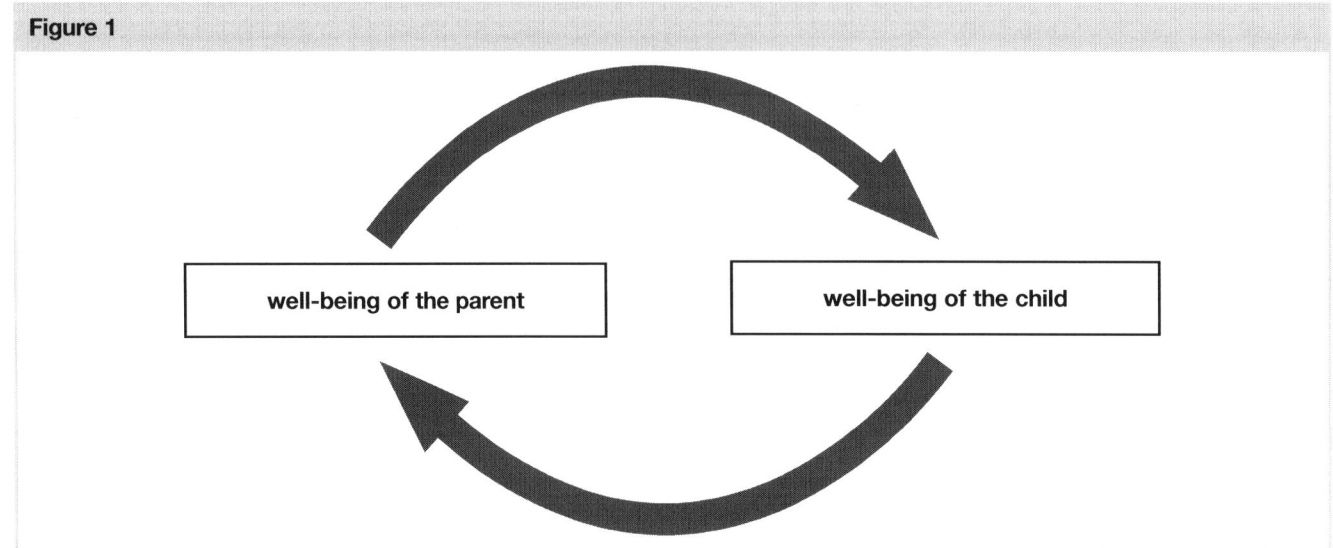

Facilitating parents to have age-appropriate conversations with children about parental mental health

Lucy and Peter came to a family liaison appointment on the inpatient ward following Lucy's admission. Peter talked about his worries for their two young children, James (four) and Matthew (two), particularly James who had been very quiet since Lucy had left the family home. It became apparent during the meeting that James believed it was his fault that Lucy was in hospital. We talked to Lucy and Peter about ways they could reassure James that it wasn't his fault. This included thinking about the language they used with James, what was said and not said in front of him, and working together to produce a simple account that James could understand.

Improving communication between all family members including children

A 17-year-old called Betty attended the family therapy clinic with her mother. Things had become so strained in their relationship that Betty had been asked to move out of the house. During our meetings we explored how cycles of arguments quickly erupted between Betty and her mum. We helped them to develop awareness of how the things they said would sound to the other person and the messages conveyed by intonation, volume and speed of speech. As a result the relationship between mother and daughter and other family members improved vastly and Betty moved back into the family home.

Promoting awareness of the well-being of the child and early warning of potential safeguarding issues

A man suffering from psychosis attended for some Family Liaison Plus sessions with his mother and his nine-year-old son. They were seen by a family therapist (Ragni) together with the patient's care co-ordinator from the community mental health team. Initially the meetings explored how the relationship between father and son functioned when dad was well and the difficulties that arose when he was unwell. It became apparent that when he was unwell he found it very difficult to set boundaries and his son, recognising this, took full advantage of it. In addition, at times when the symptoms worsened, the man struggled to cope and would then phone his mother late at night for support. During the course of these meetings, the father went through a spell of more pronounced psychosis. At this point, some separate time was given to the son and the grandmother to discuss their experience of this and to talk with the son about what was happening. The son was then able to tell us how difficult it was for him when his father became ill during these more acute episodes and this opened up some safeguarding concerns. An agreement was reached with the family (with the knowledge of the local children's safeguarding agency) that during these times of more pronounced illness the child would live with his grandmother until his father was sufficiently recovered to care for him.

Exploring the resources of the wider network

Like the previous example, this vignette also shows the importance of exploring the wider network when thinking about how mentally unwell parents can continue to parent and care for their children. Annie and her seven-year-old son, Arthur, came for a Family Liaison meeting. We explored Annie's support network and it became clear that she had some very good, long-standing friends who were very supportive to her at times of need. During this meeting, Annie became distressed as she talked about how difficult things had sometimes been for Arthur. Arthur sat and listened to his mother as she told me how she did not know what Arthur would do if she became very unwell. Arthur then reassured his mother saying, *'Well your friends would look after me of course'*. We explored this possibility and Annie acknowledged that her friends would step in and indeed had done so before. Annie agreed to make the necessary plans with these close friends.

Reconnecting families when there are disruptions in relationships

Bobby, his wife Jess, and two sons, William (16) and Luke (13), came along to a Family Liaison Plus appointment. William had physically assaulted Bobby triggering social services involvement. Since the assault, Bobby and William had not spoken, Bobby's mental health had deteriorated and the other family members were struggling with the tension in the home. The complexity and heightened emotions of the family were observed during the first meeting and we decided to separate the family in subsequent sessions. Further sessions were held with William and Luke together, and separately with Bobby and Jess. The family were then referred to family therapy with the aim of exploring ways to reconnect as a family. This included exploring what needed to happen to allow connections to be made and identifying examples of this from the past, to explore conversations around forgiveness, how they can build positive times together and what needs to happen differently in future disagreements to enable them to move forward as a family. The family therapy team provided a safe place to contain the difficult emotions, offer different perspectives and help the family to explore the circular nature of their interactions in a non-blaming way.

Identifying early warnings of child health and behavioural problems

David attended a family liaison appointment on the ward while his wife, Jessica, was an inpatient. He talked about his concerns for his children, particularly the head banging behaviour recently shown by his son, Jack, aged 10. This led to further appointments for David together with his two children during which the children were helped to understand the mental health symptoms of their mother. David was given information about monitoring any escalation in Jack's behaviour and distress.

Discussion

There may be a number of barriers to including children in adult mental health services, including:

- → not recognising the presence of children in family systems
- → children falling below service thresholds for having their own needs met
- → anxieties of professionals who feel insufficiently skilled for working with or including children
- → professionals fearing that they may impose their own parenting styles and thus usurp and disempower parents
- → professionals feeling unconfident that they are able to use child-friendly and age-appropriate ways of communicating
- → professionals feeling uncertain as to how to respond to the distress of children.

Further barriers may be presented by parents themselves, for example a reluctance to talk about their experiences of parenting for fear of losing access to their children (Ackerson, 2003; Mowbray *et al*, 1995). It is worth noting that family therapists face similar challenges when working with families where parents have mental health issues in settings other than mental health services such as family counseling services. It has been proposed that in these instances professionals need to both understand mental health issues and feel able to talk about them in therapy sessions with children (Power *et al*, 2014).

However, more recently in therapeutic settings there has been a shift away from how children are affected by parental mental health difficulties towards how parents and children can be resourced to manage these difficulties (SCIE, 2011; Krumm *et al*, 2013). We believe that helping parents to feel resourceful in relation to their own mental health and how this affects on their children can foster hope and their sense of competency despite mental health difficulties.

Furthermore, exploring the resources of the wider network in routine family inclusive practice in adult mental health services can provide safety for the children at times when parental mental health difficulties threaten the security of the parent-child relationship and the child's well-being. Having this safety net is reassuring for both parents and children, and negotiating arrangements with wider networks in advance can avoid many difficulties and misunderstandings later, reducing anxiety for all. Examples from other countries, such as Open Dialogue in Western Lapland (Seikkula, 2015) and Family Group Conferencing from New Zealand's Mauri people, have provided 'gold standard' models that are gradually being adopted within UK children's services and some adult services (see Wright, 2008).

Conclusion

In Somerset, we believe that the systemic range of work offered in adult mental health services, not only by specialists but throughout the work force, provides a vehicle for sustaining the well-being not only of the patient but of their whole family system, and a resource for recovery when implemented consistently. We have become aware that, with the introduction of Family Liaison Plus into community teams, there is an increase in both consultation and joint team working involving children. This takes into account not only the needs of the children and the needs of the unwell parent(s) but the recursive circular relationship between child and adult well-being.

We recognise the need for further training, since including children routinely in our adult services is still in its infancy, and the need for all professionals to be confident in and skilled at including children in their thinking and practice. In order to address this we are planning to include child-focused modules in future family-inclusive training for all adult mental health staff. In addition, a pilot project is being proposed that will combine ideas from art therapy with ideas from systemic family therapy to inform a group for children accompanied by carers of adult mental health patients. These plans demonstrate our ongoing thinking and work in this hitherto neglected area.

References

Ackerson BJ (2003) Coping with the dual demands of severe mental illness and parenting: the parents' perspective. *Families in Society* **84** (1) 109–119.

Beardslee WR, Versage EM & Gladstone TR (1998) Children of affectively ill parents: a review of the past 10 years. *Journal of the American Academy of Child & Adolescent Psychiatry* **37** (11) 1134–1141.

Burbach FR (2015) The development of efficient family intervention services: a whole systems approach. *Clinical Psychology Forum* (in press).

Burbach FR & Stanbridge RI (1998) A family intervention in psychosis service integrating the systemic and family management approaches. *Journal of Family Therapy* **20** (3) 311–325.

Burbach FR & Stanbridge RI (2006) Somerset's family interventions in psychosis service: an update. *Journal of Family Therapy* **28** (1) 39–57.

Cabinet Office (2008) *Think Family: Improving the life chances of families at risk* [online]. London: Social Exclusion Task Force. Available at: http://www.drugsandalcohol.ie/17766/1/think_family_life_chances_report.pdf (accessed September 2015).

Children's Society (2008) *2008 Survey* [online]. Available at http://www.childrensociety.org.uk/what-we-do/research/initiatives/well-being/background-programme/2008-survey (accessed September 2015).

Krumm S, Becker T & Weigand-Grefe S (2013) Mental health services for parents affected by mental illness. *Current Opinion in Psychiatry* **26** (4) 362–368.

Mowbray C, Oyserman D, Zemencuk JK & Ross SR (1995) Motherhood for women with serious mental illness: pregnancy, childbirth,and the postpartum period. *American Journal of Orthopsychiatry* **65** (1) 21–38.

Ofsted (2013) *What About the Children?* [online]. Available at: www.ofsted.gov.uk/resources/130066 (accessed September 2015).

Power J, Cuff R, Jewell H, McIlwaine F, O'Neill I & U'Ren G (2014) Working in a family therapy setting with families where a parent has a mental illness: practice dilemmas and strategies. *Journal of Family Therapy* DOI: 10.1111/1467-6427.12052

Seikkula J (2015) Open dialogues with clients with mental health problems and their families. *Context* **138** 2–6.

Social Care Institute for Excellence (2011) *Think Child, Think Parent, Think Family* [online]. London: SCIE. Available at http://www.scie.org.uk/publications/ataglance/ataglance09.asp (accessed September 2015).

Stanbridge R (2012) Including families and carers: an evaluation of the family liaison service on inpatient psychiatric wards in Somerset, UK. *Mental Health Review Journal* **17** (2) 70–80.

Worthington A, Rooney P & Hannan R (2013) *The Triangle of Care – Carers Included: A best practice guide in acute mental health care* (2nd edition) London: Carers Trust.

Wright T (2008) Using family group conference in mental health. *Nursing Times* **104** (4) 33–34.

Chapter 10

Early intervention to promote mental health and well-being in schools

By Dr Jane Akister and Hannah Guest

Mental health difficulties are experienced by as many as one in four people, so it could be argued that early intervention at a population, public health level is a good idea. It could also be argued that schools might be a good setting for early intervention, if we had evidence that it works. This chapter proposes that child mental health is a vital element of overall child well-being, discusses the concept of early intervention, looks at early intervention strategies and presents research findings that suggest that the reasons behind the lack of concrete evidence of effective early intervention to promote and protect young people (Licence, 2004) is that a schools-based, targeted approach is needed.

Parents with any combination of mental health, substance abuse or experiences of domestic violence are known to be linked to child protection issues (Brandon *et al*, 2010). Parents who have mental health problems are therefore understandably reluctant to seek help with parenting, for fear of the consequences for their family. We also know that poor mental health at 16 years old is a significant determinant for poor mental health outcomes into adulthood (Case *et al*, 2005). Consequences of poor mental health include lower educational attainment, poorer health and lower social status as adults.

To fully understand early intervention and the effects it can have, there are a number of questions to be considered:

→ When is it most effective?

→ Why is it effective? What are the outcomes, how are they measured and proved to have causality with the outcome and the project?

→ Who should receive the intervention? Should it be available for everyone (universal)? Should only the 'at risk' receive the intervention (targeted)?

→ What setting should early intervention be in?

→ Who should and could be delivering programmes of early intervention?

→ How can prevention programmes and intervention engage the people they are intended for?

→ Is early intervention cost effective compared to the alternatives of no intervention or more traditional support?

Statham and Smith (2010) discuss the difference between support and intervention, proposing that all interventions should be experienced by children and families as something they are included in and that they really do feel is in their best interest. The concept of intervention suggests that something needs to change. For example, if a child is behaving badly in school then an intervention could take the form of working with the child to better develop their coping skills and help them to understand why the behaviour is not allowed. Both rely on helping the child to change their current behaviour. In this same case, support would look different. Once the child had a strategy to change their behaviour or regulate their impulses, then support could be allowing the child more time to process situations or making sure they have additional support in upsetting circumstances to enable them to cope.

In the case of early intervention, the distinction between intervention and support becomes less clear. To commission an early intervention for people who do not currently meet thresholds for services but perhaps are at risk of doing so in the future, there needs to be evidence that the outcomes of the intervention are going to be positive. Did the intervention provide a positive outcome in terms of educational attainment or reducing crime or reducing the prevalence of depression in adolescents? Did the intervention provide a good economic outcome for wider society? These are just a few questions that highlight how difficult it is to evidence effectiveness for early intervention even though intuitively it seems like a good idea.

Universal or targeted intervention?

A key question for early intervention is whether it should be universal or targeted. Universal interventions are popular because they do not stigmatise or label anyone, but they can be very costly. A universal intervention has potential when used within an existing setting, for example a school, and several different school projects have shown that all children can benefit from an intervention. A well designed school-based intervention could benefit a large population of children and tackle a common problem with high prevalence, and this could be implemented within a pre-scheduled class, such as PSHE (personal, social, health and economic education), which already provides work around well-being. Children in this situation are essentially a 'captive audience'. Research indicates that teachers can be trained to provide mental well-being programmes as effectively as trained mental health professionals (Collins *et al*, 2013).

Targeted interventions, meanwhile, focus on children identified to be 'at risk', such as The Scallywags programme in Cornwall which targets children who have been referred with signs of conduct problems (Broadhead *et al*, 2009). It can be argued that it is important to build an evidence base for the positive effects of early intervention targeted on emerging problems.

A model of intervention increasingly favoured by government is 'progressive universalism'. Progressive universalism offers basic public health services to everyone and then offers specific specialised services to those most at risk.

Identifying those at risk and who may need early intervention

Accurately identifying children who are at risk is difficult. For instance, according to evidence and research, children whose parents have mental health problems are at risk of various negative outcomes, however, clearly not all children will be affected. A child who has more than one characteristic that may be considered a risk becomes more likely to suffer harm and the risk of potential harm becomes greater (Bynner, 2001). When parents raise concerns, professionals need to hear what help they are asking for and ensure they start their work at the point where there are risks and signs of harm but before the family reach a crisis. Within the Scallywags early intervention programme, in order for a child to be accepted onto the programme they have to have a referral from both a care giver and a professional who has contact with the child. If the professional does not see a high enough level of risk in the conduct of the child, there is potential that they will be missed out and there is a risk that parents will not engage with services again when they need help.

We know of cases in which children could have been saved from significant harm if initial reports of concern or seeking help had been responded to by the appropriate agency, but early intervention and prevention work must not be seen as a substitute for traditional services that provide support and intervention to those who, for instance, need immediate help to deal with a crisis.

Do early interventions work?

Reviewing early interventions designed to prevent depression in young people, Merry and Spence (2007) found no evidence that universal interventions worked in schools to reduce depression. However, while there were minimal benefits in relation to depressive symptoms, they did find other benefits, such as a reduction in anxiety or improvements in self-esteem and confidence, although they warn that there is not enough evidence to prove that early intervention should be implemented more widely.

Lubans *et al* (2012) reviewed activity projects that are designed to promote social and emotional well-being in children who have been identified as at risk. Their review concluded that 'outdoor' activity programmes had the most positive effects, including improved resilience, self-concept, self-perceptions, perceived physical competence and mood regulation. It was unclear, however, what elements of outdoor activities were most effective at creating these positive outcomes, and of the 15 programmes reviewed there were four that had no effect on the children when compared to a control group. This is important to remember when discussing early intervention, as it is possible to assume that any form of programme designed to promote well-being will have some benefits.

Another element of early intervention is its timing. Programmes that appear effective with pre-secondary school children do not necessarily work with older children. Gillham *et al* (1995) implemented a school-based intervention model to teach children aged between 10 and 11 years old skills to reduce their depressive symptoms. Positive results are reported for reducing depressive symptoms and learning coping strategies, which were maintained on follow-up. Roberts *et al* (2003) used the same model of intervention with 12-year-old children in Australia but had very different results. This shows how problematic evidence surrounding early intervention can be, as there is often little generalisability between very similar projects.

In the UK, Scallywags is a good example of a targeted intervention project designed to help children identified as having conduct problems (Broadhead *et al*, 2009). The project's 411 students received a six-month intervention both at school and home, using family support workers to improve behaviour and help parents to reduce conduct problems. Teachers and parent reports indicated 60% of those who were within clinical range for conduct disorders were in the normal range after intervention. Parents reported that the Scallywags programme had a significant impact on their lives and their children's behaviour. The report doesn't contain evidence of long-term follow up data, but as Scallywags was a highly intense and expensive programme, it is important to know if the results were sustained.

One of the benefits of universal intervention is that it gives the potential for people to receive help who may not have been identified as needing it. An Australian programme provided an intervention to a whole school population aiming to reduce adolescent depression (Shochet *et al*, 2001). Two-hundred and sixty 14-year-old children were randomly allocated to three groups: just adolescents, adolescents and parents, and a control group just for adolescents. Both intervention groups showed positive results for depressive symptoms compared to the control group, however there was no significant difference between the two groups, making it difficult to know which intervention worked most effectively. Recruitment was high, which is a common benefit to using universal interventions.

Other programmes using cognitive behavioural therapy (CBT) with children in schools have reported positive results, including CBT with nine to ten year olds (Collins *et al*, 2013), and CBT with 13 year olds in America (Puskar *et al*, 1999). School-based interventions are easier to implement and less costly to run than those based in the community, but evidence for the sustainability of effects is vital before rolling out such interventions. We should also be mindful that so far there is not enough evidence to implement early intervention more widely.

Interventions to prepare children for secondary school

The transition between primary and secondary school has been identified as an important point in childhood that can be very difficult for some children (Evangelou et al, 2008). Several summer school projects have aimed to help children with the transition, but while the results are promising, the research again suffers from being small in scale with fairly minimal outcomes. Rock Up, although a small Australian project with no control group, did show how work can be done with children at risk to improve their experience of this important transition (Carmen et al, 2011). The project worked with 13 children who were aged ten and who were identified by teachers as being at risk of disengaging from formal education as they started secondary school. The children either had individual time with a support worker or group activities to facilitate the transition and promote well-being. The support workers also worked with their parents to help them learn skills to support their child with the transition. While the sample is small, the results are interesting. The students reported feeling more confident and less worried about the transition. Parents also said that their children seemed to get a lot out of the intervention and that they enjoyed it. The qualitative data collected showed that there was improvement from pre-intervention to post-intervention. The reported benefits were not sustained on the follow up and this is a common problem in early intervention programs. Sustained results would be necessary to make it worthwhile, in cost terms, to adopt any programme involving work within the school and at home.

Martin et al (2013) surveyed 21,065 students who went to summer schools or who were in comparison schools. The majority of the data collected centred on whether the children enjoyed the summer school and whether they felt more prepared for their secondary school. The vast majority of schools and children considered the summer school a success and the students found them enjoyable. Students said that they felt more prepared for the transition and less worried about attending, but it is unclear whether they actually had a smoother transition because of the summer school, even though the children thought they would. The study found that, of those invited, more girls than boys took part in the summer school, and that those from an Asian background were less likely to attend if invited. While 83% of those who were invited did attend the summer school, it is important to remember that some children who were identified as being from disadvantaged backgrounds did not. The children who do not attend universal programmes may well be those who could potentially benefit the most.

Another summer school aimed to ensure that children from disadvantaged backgrounds did not experience a reduction of numeracy and literacy skills over the summer. This summer school consisted of numeracy and literacy classes in the morning and activities in the afternoon. There were no significant differences between the intervention group and control data and both groups experienced a loss in skills in numeracy and literacy over the summer (Siddiqu et al, 2014). 'Summer loss' is common for children, and these results are disappointing. This study is a good example of how early interventions are not guaranteed to have positive results simply because the funding and execution was implemented. It is very hard to design a universal programme that is likely to match with the participants' needs.

East Cambridgeshire and Fenland Project

Our research in East Cambridgeshire and Fenland was at the invitation of the Cambridgeshire Children's Trust, who were concerned about children disengaging with education on transition to secondary school (Akister, 2014). The research we undertook was designed to look at the mental well-being of children aged 10–11 years old, just before their transition to secondary school. Ten primary schools were involved in the study, feeding into two comprehensive secondary schools.

For each child that the teachers were concerned about (n=48), the teachers were asked to complete a strengths and difficulties questionnaire (SDQ) and identify the reasons for their concern. Following this, the students were offered transitions projects over the school summer holidays and then repeat SDQs were completed by the students' tutors at the end of their first year at secondary school. Consent was sought from all parents whose children were identified as in need of additional support in the transition.

Factors that can be linked to poor educational attainment include negative school experiences, lack of self-confidence and self-esteem, and persistent truancy, although the causes of truancy have not been significantly researched (Sachdev et al, 2006). From Table 1 we can see that 48% of the children scored high for overall stress scores on the SDQ, with the subscales emotional distress scoring highly. The change in the overall stress scores (from 48% to 13%) and emotional distress scores (from 40% to 15%) pre- and post-summer activity project suggest the effectiveness of the project, specifically in the domains of self-confidence and self-esteem, known to be important for educational attainment.

Table 1: East Cambridgeshire and Fenland Project SDQ scores

	Pre-secondary school scores	End of first year at secondary school scores
Overall stress	48%	13%
Emotional distress	40%	15%
Hyperactivity	42%	41%
Behavioural difficulties	23%	18%

For some of the children, behavioural difficulties and hyperactivity are the major reasons for concern. Table 1 indicates that there was little change in the subscales of the SDQ relating to behaviour: hyperactivity (from 42% to 41%); behavioural difficulties (from 23% to 18%). This project supports the approach of targeting activity projects on specific needs, as the well-being of those children with emotional distress is greatly improved, and maintained over a 12-month period, whereas for those children with behavioural difficulties, no significant improvement is sustained. It is interesting that the measure of well-being gives such a clear indication of the success of the project, and this suggests that the design of the project, which aimed at improving self-confidence and peer relationships, is effective.

That such a project is not successful at improving behaviour suggests that we should not place all the children who are of concern in the same project. A universal project aimed at helping with the transition will have mixed results if all children are included. Specific projects targeted at behaviour are needed in addition to those promoting self-confidence.

Conclusion

The mental well-being of young people is a major factor in the educational outcomes they are able to achieve and in their life opportunities. Early intervention projects are very attractive as we can identify children with difficulties quite early in the educational process, but the evidence to support universal 'one size fits all' interventions is very mixed. Our research in East Cambridgeshire and Fenland suggests that teachers are accurate in identifying young people with poor mental well-being and that this includes two main groups: those with emotional distress (internalising) and those with behavioural difficulties (externalising). If targeted 'early intervention' approaches are taken focusing on either of these, we suggest that the outcomes will be much more positive than in those projects where everyone is offered the same universal early intervention.

References

Akister J (2014) *Outcomes After a Year at Secondary School for Students Identified as in Need of Additional Support in the Transition from Primary School: Report for Cambridgeshire Children's Trust.* Anglia Ruskin Publications.

Brandon M, Bailey S & Belderson P (2010) *Building on the Learning from Serious Case Reviews: A two-year analysis of child protection database notifications 2007-2009* [online]. London: Department for Education. Available at: https://www.gov.uk/government/uploads/system/uploads/attachment_data/file/181651/DFE-RR040.pdf (accessed September 2015).

Broadhead MA, Hockaday A, Zahra M, Francis PJ & Crichton C (2009) Scallywags: an evaluation of a service targeting conduct disorders at school and at home. *Educational Psychology in Practice* **25** (2) 167–179.

Bynner J (2001) Childhood risks and protective factors in social exclusion. *Children & Society* **15** (5) 285-301.

Carmen B, Waycott L & Smith K (2011) Rock Up: an initiative supporting students' wellbeing in their transition to secondary school. *Children and Youth Services Review* **33** (1) 167–172.

Case A, Fertig A & Paxson C (2005) The lasting impact of childhood health and circumstance. *Journal of Health Economics* **24** (2) 365–389.

Collins S, Woolfson LM & Durkin K (2013) Effects on coping skills and anxiety of a universal school-based mental health intervention delivered in Scottish primary schools. *School Psychology International* doi: 10.1177/0143034312469157.

Evangelou, M (2008) *What Makes a Successful Transition from Primary to Secondary School?* [online]. Available at: http://dera.ioe.ac.uk/8618/7/DCSF-RB019.pdf (accessed September 2015).

Gillham JE, Reivich KJ, Jaycox LH & Seligman ME (1995) Prevention of depressive symptoms in schoolchildren: two-year follow-up. *Psychological Science* **6** (6) 343–351.

Licence K (2004) Promoting and protecting the health of children and young people. *Childcare, Health and Development* **30** (6) 623–635.

Lubans DR, Plotnikoff RC & Lubans NJ (2012) Review: a systematic review of the impact of physical activity programmes on social and emotional wellbeing in at-risk youth. *Child and Adolescent Mental Health* **17** (1) 2–13.

Martin K, Sharp C & Mehta P (2013) *The Impact of the Summer Schools Programme on Pupils* [online]. Slough: National Foundation for Education Research. Available at: https://www.nfer.ac.uk/publications/ESSP04/ESSP04_home.cfm (accessed September 2015).

Merry SN & Spence SH (2007) Attempting to prevent depression in youth: a systematic review of the evidence. *Early Intervention in Psychiatry* **1** (2) 128–137.

Puskar KR, Sereika SM, Lamb J, Tusaie-Mumford K & Mcguinness T (1999) Optimism and its relationship to depression, coping, anger, and life events in rural adolescents. *Issues in Mental Health Nursing* **20** (2) 115–130.

Roberts C, Kane R, Thomson H, Bishop B & Hart B (2003) The prevention of depressive symptoms in rural school children: a randomized controlled trial. *Journal of Consulting and Clinical Psychology* **71** (3) 622.

Sachdev D, Harries B & Roberts T (2006) *Regional and Sub-regional Variation in NEETs–Reasons, Remedies and Impact* [online]. Learning and Skills Development Agency. Available at: http://s3.amazonaws.com/zanran_storage/www.yorkshirefutures.com/ContentPages/1272832320.pdf (accessed September 2015).

Shochet IM, Dadds MR, Holland D, Whitefield K, Harnett PH & Osgarby SM (2001) The efficacy of a universal school-based program to prevent adolescent depression. *Journal of Clinical Child Psychology* **30** (3) 303–315.

Siddiqui N, Gorard S & See BH (2014) Is a summer school programme a promising intervention in preparation for transition from primary to secondary school? *International Education Studies* **7** (7) 125.

Statham J & Smith M (2010) *Issues in Earlier Intervention: Identifying and supporting children with additional needs.* Institute of Education, University of London: Thomas Coram Research Unit.

Chapter 11

School children's vulnerability audit tool

By Wendy Weal

There is a great opportunity for schools and early years providers following the Department for Communities and Local Government's (DCLG) announcement that there will be more funding put towards helping vulnerable children and families through the expansion of the troubled families programme. Few could argue that helping children and families at an earlier stage is the right way to move forward.

We know that schools and early years providers know who these families are. Ask a reception teacher about their children and they will know from a young age who the children are who are likely to go on to have long-term behavioural difficulties. These are the children who, when older, are more likely to truant and be excluded, and possibly commit anti-social behaviour and crime. But do school staff think about this proactively and do something with that information? Or do they just react when they need to?

We believe that the only effective way to achieve positive outcomes for children is to think about and work with the wider family. We know that growing up in a family with significant social, health, economic and behavioural problems has a lasting and inter-generational impact on a child's life chances. We also know that around 120,000 families in England experience multiple social, health and economic problems and 46,000 of these experience 'problem' child behaviour (ODPM, 2004). In terms of schooling they account for a large number of school exclusions and one fifth of youth offences (ODPM, 2004). Their parents are 34 times more likely to need drug treatment, eight times more likely to need alcohol treatment and a third of their children are subject to child protection (ODPM, 2004).

We also know that effective parenting can protect against the effects and risks of growing up in a poor or deprived neighbourhood, and reduce the likelihood of anti-social behaviour and crime. The impacts on educational attainment are particularly well documented. For instance, we know that parental interest in education is four times more important than other social and economic factors in influencing attainment at 16 and that parental involvement in education has a bigger impact on attainment at seven and 11 than the quality of the school, even controlling for social class (Cabinet Office, 2008).

So, if we know the factors that lead to poor outcomes, there is a strong argument for schools and academies proactively considering the needs of the children and their families in order to support them to achieve better outcomes in terms of life chances as well as with their academic attainment.

We have therefore worked with schools to develop an electronic tool, the Schools' Vulnerable Children Audit Tool, to help senior leadership teams, teachers, support staff and multi-agency partners to identify vulnerable children and their families and work more effectively and efficiently with them.

We saw a need for this after our work with schools showed a need for them to consider questions about, and work with, the wider family and community when supporting any child. We also saw situations where schools were 'holding' high-need cases and not receiving enough support from multi-agency partners. But, overwhelmingly, we observed schools not knowing and not asking questions about what was going on in a child's life outside the school gates – their wider environment.

Very timely, therefore, was the release of the Department for Education's Family Stressors research (Jones et al, 2013), which provides clear evidence that children can experience a range of stressful situations which lead to potential vulnerability with respect to their educational development and well-being.

The findings are helpful in flagging up the areas where children may be at risk of failing badly on educational and well-being outcomes, and where interventions (by schools working in partnership with other agencies) might be justifiably targeted to help to close 'achievement gaps'. The research tells us there is a direct link between vulnerability and attainment or achievement of children. But we know that converting that knowledge into strategies and interventions is difficult, and tracking the impact of those strategies and interventions is a further challenge. We therefore incorporated all the factors identified in the research as having a clear impact on children's educational achievement into our children's school vulnerability audit tool.

The tool looks in depth at the individual child's vulnerability. What do we know about their health, social development, family, social relationships, self-care, parent's attitude and engagement, housing etc.? We talk to special education needs co-ordinator (SENCO) leads who are not asking these questions, often stating issues of time constraints, however this understanding is crucial in order to effectively support a child and stop issues escalating. When we look at serious case reviews or map a family's journey we will see 'trigger points' where we could have intervened earlier but didn't and see the negative results of this. We must look at this proactively and not reactively, given all that research tells us.

Schools work through a detailed 'holistic' analysis using a range of indicators of the potential vulnerability of individual children.

Figure 1 shows the areas that the tool covers in depth.

Figure 1: Scope of the Schools' Vulnerable Children Audit Tool

Physical, emotional and social development	Health
	Emotional/social development
	Behavioural development
	Self esteem/image
	Family and social relationships
	Self care and independence
Learning and schooling	Attendance, punctuality, moves
	Learning, achievement and attainment
	Additional educational needs
	Social relationships and behaviour
	Parent's attitudes and engagement
Parents and carers	Basic care, safety and protection
	Emotional warmth and stability
	Guidance, boundaries and stimulation
The wider family and community	Wider family
	Housing/financial considerations
	Social and community resources

Users can record the actions/interventions that they have put into place to help mitigate the effects of the vulnerability factors, and importantly record the impact of those actions/interventions – crucial to consider what works, why and when, and, of course, it is also good to demonstrate to Ofsted.

The tool aggregates the individual pupil vulnerability profiles to provide a cohort or school-level picture of the vulnerability of children across the school so that decisions can be made about resource allocations and group-level interventions. This means that resources can be effectively targeted.

It also shows quickly where there are gaps in knowledge, and this is where multi-agency partners come in. What do they jointly know about the wider family, their community etc.? Schools should work with partners to consider in some depth the challenges an individual child is facing and how best to put in place mitigating actions/interventions. But, importantly, they can also share concerns across the partnership based on what the whole school data is showing. Is there a group of year eight girls self-harming, for example? Are there concerns that

a high percentage of children are caring for parents with mental health issues? We know that in a class of 26 primary school children, six or seven children are living with a mother with mental health difficulties (Layard, 2005; Meltzer et al, 2000). We also know that of the 175,000 young carers identified in the 2001 census, 29% (just over 50,000) are estimated to care for a family member with mental health difficulties (ODPM, 2004). Schools therefore need to know who they are and consider, with partners, how to best support them.

The tool is used both as an individual planning tool for a child and as a strategic planning tool to make decisions across the school and the partnership. It also provides an evidence base for both Ofsted inspections (schools can demonstrate that they know their children and can demonstrate the impact of interventions) and for generating a more informed discussion to support collaborative working with partner organisations. A typical finding is that children and adolescent mental health services (CAMHs) are not responsive enough to meet the needs in schools. Anecdotal evidence suggests that many schools feel frustrated that their children's mental health needs are not being met and the tool provides the evidence for this. This generates a local conversation for multi-agency partners to demonstrate local need and consider how best to support this with mitigating actions/interventions.

The potential to support children in a more proactive way is massive. Everyone has increasingly tight budgets. Reacting at crisis points is not cheap nor a long-term workable solution. We need to 'think family, think community and think proactively' to bring about sustainable improvements in the lives of vulnerable children.

You can find out more about the school vulnerability tool by calling 01603 251730 or by visiting www.interfaceenterprises.co.uk

References

Cabinet Office (2008) *Think Family: Improving the life chances of families at risk*. London: Cabinet Office Social Exclusion Unit.

Jones E, Gutman L & Platt L (2013) *Family Stressors and Outcomes* [online]. London: Department for Education. Available at: https://www.gov.uk/government/publications/family-stressors-and-childrens-outcomes (accessed September 2015).

Layard R (2005) *Mental Health: Britain's biggest social problem?* [online] In: Paper presented at the No.10 Strategy Unit Seminar on Mental Health, 20th January 2005, London, UK. Available at: http://eprints.lse.ac.uk/47428/ (accessed September 2015).

Meltzer H, Gatward R, Goodman R & Ford T (2000) *The Mental Health of Children and Adolescents in Great Britain* London: Office for National Statistics.

ODPM (2004) *Mental Health and Social Exclusion: Social Exclusion Unit report* [online]. London: Office of the Deputy Prime Minister. Available at: http://tse.two-seas.eu/filelib/file/mentalhealthsocialexclusion.pdf (accessed September 2015).

Impacts and influences on mental health recovery, parenting and children's development and well-being

Chapter 12

Parental mental health and young carers: children (and families) first

By Professor Jo Aldridge

It has been 12 years since findings were published from the first ever research in the UK on the impacts on children of caring for parents with mental illness (Aldridge & Becker, 2003). Since that time, 'young carers' have been identified in newly implemented policy and practice and, at the time of writing, a new national study is underway to more accurately identify the numbers of children in England who provide care for parents with illness/disability[1].

Despite these advances, the 2003 study remains the only one of its kind to date to provide estimates of the numbers of children caring for parents with mental health problems specifically. Taking a triangulated approach, the study included the views of children, the parents for whom they were providing care and the professionals involved in delivering health and social care services to these families.

In the last decade or so, there has been a notable shift in mental health policy and practice, away from a strictly patient-led approach to assessing and meeting the needs of adults affected by mental illness towards family-based models of working, which also consider parenting needs and the importance of children's involvement in care planning decisions, needs assessments and so on. In recent years, this shift has been underscored, both philosophically and in practice, by a move away from a strictly medical model to a social model of mental illness.

This is also reflected in the emergence and advancement of the parental mental health and child welfare paradigm, that attempts to ensure the views of children, parents and families are at the forefront of mental health service delivery. In the UK, this has manifested in new family-based policies and models of working with adults who have mental health problems and who are also parents. For example, the 'Think Family' programme (Department for Children, Schools and Families, 2009), *Think Child, Think Parent, Think Family* guidance (Social Care Institute for Excellence, 2012) and government policies and initiatives that have included, for example, *No Health without Mental Health* (HM Government, 2011) and *Troubled Families* (Department for Communities and Local Government, 2012).

While it is undoubtedly the case that the young carers' paradigm has been influential in promoting children's rights – including their rights to needs assessments as carers, and to participation and consultation (including being involved in care planning decisions) – it is also clear that there have been, and remain, limitations to the somewhat narrow or circumscribed dimensions of the young carer paradigm; specifically, its somewhat exclusive focus on children's (caring) roles and responsibilities in the context of family illness/disability, including parental mental illness.

As is embodied within the parental mental health and child welfare paradigm (and congruent also with family-based models of intervention), caring should be considered as just one of the consequences for children of living in families affected by parental mental illness, and especially when parents are not provided with the necessary health, social care and parenting support to meet all of their needs. Thus, it is important to consider children in these contexts as children first, rather than simply as carers. Furthermore, while parental mental illness can be an indicator or trigger for the onset of caring among children, it should not be considered an inevitable outcome of such, and it is important that health and social care professionals recognise this. In order to ensure that children are not drawn into inappropriate caring roles when parents experience mental health problems, what are needed are early, family-based interventions (that take into account the needs of adults with mental health problems, their parenting needs and the needs of their children) at the point of onset (see Aldridge & Becker, 2003; Aldridge, 2006).

Currently in the UK, guidance for professionals (in both adult and children's services) who work with families affected by parental mental illness is somewhat diverse, but delineated by the different agendas of two separate (albeit not unrelated) perspectives: the broader family perspective on parental mental health, with its locus in the parental mental health and child welfare paradigm (where children are considered first as children, and not as carers); and the young carers paradigm, with its somewhat narrower focus on children's roles and responsibilities and the impact of these on their lives (carers first).

The distinction between these two approaches can be seen in the different emphasis placed on children's needs and the

---

[1] *Young Carers in England* is a national study funded by the Department for Education that started in September 2014 and is due for completion April 2016.

needs of families in mental health guidance for health and social care professionals who work with families affected by parental mental illness. For example, guidance from SCIE (2015) frames parental mental illness as a child and family welfare issue and highlights the importance of professional roles in implementing and working within 'family' threshold criteria for access to services to take into account the individual and combined needs of parents, carers and children. Strategies for the management of joint cases should be recorded where the situation is complex or there is a high risk of poor outcomes for children and parents' (see also Evans & Fowler, 2008).

In contrast, guidance for professionals produced by the Children's Society (2011) identifies children in families where parental mental illness is present primarily as carers, and the challenges they face originating from their need to provide care:

> 'Families who are unsupported in these situations may find it difficult to cope and sometimes rely on children to take on inappropriate caring responsibilities. This can impact on the child's physical health, emotional wellbeing and future prospects.' (p2)

Effective needs assessments for children who live in families affected by mental illness should consider the needs of adults (as patients, service users and as parents) and the needs of children not simply or mainly as carers. Other issues are likely to be equally, or more, important: for example, the emotional impact on children of having a parent with a mental illness, the impact on children's education, their transitions into adulthood, relationships with parents, peers and so on, as well as the role of significant others in families' lives. Alongside these, children's own mental health issues (and risks) should also be considered. This is especially significant given that recent evidence shows a marked increase in emotional problems in young people, and particularly among girls – for example, a 2015 study conducted by academics from University College London and the Anna Freud Centre found that, 'emotional problems in girls aged 11-13 in England increased by 55% between 2009 and 2014' (Fink et al, 2015).

The need to locate (or relocate) the needs of children in families affected by parental mental illness outside the narrow (micro) confines of the young carer paradigm – so that they are considered and assessed as children first rather than as carers – is also demonstrated in broader (macro) perspectives on the effects on families of systemic dynamics. Research evidence on the effects of low income and poverty in families, for example, has shown how these circumstances can transform children's roles and responsibilities within families. Tess Ridge's 2009 research, for example, showed that:

> '...children in low-income working families were often taking on additional responsibilities in the home, including housework and caring responsibilities, or engaged in paid work themselves to ease financial pressures at home and to gain access to their own money' (p 4).

This approach identifies and locates child caring as a consequence of the effects of poverty and austerity in families, rather than simply as an inevitable consequence of parental illness/disability.

The need for professionals to understand and assess the parenting needs of adults who experience mental illness as well as the needs of their children (including their caring needs), was a significant feature of our research findings and recommendations in the 2003 mental health research, and later studies on young carers and their families (see Dearden & Aldridge, 2010). However, outside the mental health field, it is still the case that some health and social care professionals who work with young carers and their families remain unclear about how to conduct needs assessments using a family-based approach. The introduction of new policy and guidance in the form of the Care Act (2014) and the Children and Families Act (2014) (HM Government, 2014a; 2014b), attempts to remedy both the piecemeal and inconsistent nature of previous policy (and practice) on young carers, as well as address the lack of clarity about how professionals can make effective family-based assessments. Notably, the Children and Families Act (2014) makes amendments to the Children Act (1989) to include young carers' needs assessments. However, importantly, it maintains emphasis on their wider needs as children, referring (in section 17ZA (7)) to the need for assessments to establish, 'whether it is appropriate for the young carer to provide, or continue to provide, care for the person in question, in the light of the young carer's needs for support, other needs and wishes'. Further, in section 17ZA (11), the act goes on to state, 'where the person cared for is under 18, the written record must state whether the local authority consider him or her to be a child in need.'

One of the key messages to emerge from the 2003 mental health study that continues to be a challenge today regarding the implementation of family-based interventions is that children (and parents) are often afraid to disclose caring responsibilities – and the further impacts on children of living with parent with mental illness – through fear of safeguarding or child protection decisions that might lead to family separations. Such fears are perhaps not unrealistic given the rise in the number of children placed in local authority care as a result of parental illness/disability – in 2013 (House of Commons, 2014) 2,500 children were admitted to local authority care. Other reasons included 'family stress', 'neglect' 'absent parenting' and 'socially unacceptable behaviour' (and together accounted for more than 50,000 children being admitted into local authority care). Some or all of these factors may be pertinent in families affected by parental mental illness when parents, children and families do not receive the kind of assessments and support services they need.

Other messages from the 2003 research that were also mirrored in mental health research and recommendations around that time (see Falkov, 1998), have since been identified as critical in ensuring that the parenting needs of adults with mental illness and the needs of families are met effectively. As is stated in SCIE's 2015 guidance, professionals need to:

> 'routinely and reliably identify and record information about which adults with mental health problems are parents, and which children have parents with mental health problems. This means developing systems and tools in collaboration with parents and young people, to ensure the right questions are asked and the data is recorded for future use.' (SCIE, 2015).

In summary, while putting the spotlight on young carers in research, policy and practice has undoubtedly helped to transform the lives of many families where parental illness (including mental illness) or disability is present, children's caring responsibilities should not be the sole focus of health and social care interventions aimed at helping families. For many children and young people, an increase in caring responsibilities will be just one of the outcomes of living in families where parents experience illness/disability and, like other outcomes for children in these contexts, these are more likely to be problematic and lead to adverse consequences for children when the parenting needs of adults, and the needs of children and families, are not met.

References

Aldridge J (2006) The experiences of children living with and caring for parents with mental illness. *Child Abuse Review* **15** (2) 79–88.

Aldridge J & Becker S (2003) *Children Caring for Parents With Mental Illness: Perspectives of young carers, parents and professionals.* Bristol: The Policy Press.

Children's Society (2011) *Supporting Children Who Have a Parent With a Mental Illness: Information for professionals* [online]. Available at: http://www.youngcarer.com/sites/default/files/mental_illness_booklet_2011_2nd.pdf (accessed September 2015).

Dearden CM & Aldridge J (2010) Young carers: Needs, rights and assessment. In: J Horwath *The child's world: Assessing children in need* (2nd edition). London: Jessica Kingsley.

Department for Children, Schools and Families (2009) *Think Family Toolkit: Improving support for families at risk: Strategic overview* [online]. Available at: http://webarchive.nationalarchives.gov.uk/20130401151715/http://www.education.gov.uk/publications/eOrderingDownload/Think-Family.pdf (accessed September 2015).

Department for Communities and Local Government (2012) *Troubled Families Programme* [online]. Available at: https://www.gov.uk/government/policies/helping-troubled-families-turn-their-lives-around (accessed September 2015).

Evans J & Fowler R (2008) *Family Minded: Supporting children in families affected by mental illness* [online]. London: Barnardos. Available at: http://www.barnardos.org.uk/family_minded_report.pdf (accessed September 2015).

Falkov A (1998) *Crossing Bridges: Training resources for working with mentally ill parents and their children.* London: Department of Health.

Fink E, Patalay P, Sharpe H, Holley S, Deighton J & Wolpert M (2015) Mental health difficulties in early adolescence: a comparison of two cross-sectional studies in England from 2009 to 2014. *Journal of Adolescent Health* **56** (5) 502–507.

HM Government (2011) *No Health Without Mental Health: A cross-government mental health outcomes strategy for people of all ages* [online]. Available at: https://www.gov.uk/government/uploads/system/uploads/attachment_data/file/213761/dh_124058.pdf (accessed September 2015).

HM Government (2014a) *Care Act* (2014) [online]. Available at: http://www.legislation.gov.uk/ukpga/2014/23/contents/enacted (accessed September 2015).

HM Government (2014b) *Children and Families Act* (2014) [online]. Available at: http://www.legislation.gov.uk/ukpga/2014/6/section/96/enacted?view=plain (accessed September 2015).

House of Commons (2014) *Children in Care in England: Statistics* [online]. Available at: www.parliament.uk/briefing-papers/sn04470.pdf (accessed September 2015).

Ridge T (2009) *Living With Poverty: A review of the literature on children's and families' experiences of poverty – Research Report number 594.* London: Department for Work and Pensions.

SCIE (2012) *Think Child, Think Parent, Think Family.* London: Social Care Institute for Excellence.

SCIE (2015) *Parental Mental Health and Child Welfare: A guide for adult and children's health and social care services* [online]. Available at: http://www.scie.org.uk/publications/guides/guide30/assessment.asp (accessed September 2015).

Chapter 13

Fathers with mental health problems: challenging stigma, promoting inclusion

By Rhys Price-Robertson and Associate Professor Andrea Reupert

Introduction

Parents with mental health problems must negotiate all the joys and challenges of parenthood, while simultaneously managing the symptoms of their ill-health. Unfortunately, such parents often face the judgemental and disapproving reactions of others, especially in regard to their capacity to provide appropriate care to their children. This chapter will focus on the experiences of fathers with mental health problems and the specific forms of stigma they face.

A recent review explored the detrimental role that mental illness stigma can play in the lives of fathers and their families (Price-Robertson et al, in press). Although *'the stigmatisation that surrounds mental illness is increasingly recognised as a central issue, if not the central issue, for the entire mental health field'* (Hinshaw, 2005, p 714), this review was the first to focus specifically on the stigma experiences of fathers with mental health problems. This chapter will outline some of the key findings from this review, and further explore the implications these findings may have for managers, practitioners and policymakers working in health and social care. We focus on two issues: the impact stigma may have on fathers' help-seeking behaviours, and the forms of stigma that may be perpetuated by various human service sectors, in particular the child welfare sector. At the end of each section, we provide practice reflections, designed to encourage readers to consider the ways in which mental illness stigma may influence their professional activities, as well as the lives of the families they work with.

Fathers and mental illness stigma

Stigma can be broadly defined as a *'…global devaluation of certain individuals on the basis of some characteristic they possess, related to membership in a group that is disfavoured, devalued, or disgraced by the general society'* (Hinshaw, 2005, p23). Many in the community perceive those with mental health problems as deviant, incompetent, different, dangerous and/or undesirable (Phelan, 2005). Moreover, when people with mental health problems become parents, they are subject to new responsibilities, expectations and norms, and so the stigma they face can take new forms. For instance, parents may be judged as dangerous or incompetent – unable to fulfil the responsibilities expected of them as parents – based solely on their mental health status.

Most of the existing research on parenting and mental illness stigma has focused on mothers, or has included a large majority of mothers in a mixed-sex sample and failed to distinguish potential gender differences (Price-Robertson, 2015). There are many possible reasons for this, including the perception that parenting is more relevant to women than to men, and women's higher prevalence rates for some of the most common psychological disorders (Elgar et al, 2007). We believe that it is important to distinguish fathers' experiences, as men may experience mental health problems differently to women, often use different strategies to self-manage health problems, and are subject to different gender and parenting social norms than women (Price-Robertson, 2015).

Price-Robertson et al (in press) examined available qualitative research on the experiences of fathers with mental health problems, with a particular focus on how stigma was discussed in this literature. Occurrences of stigma were coded using Pryor and Reeder's (2011) four-part typology of stigma i.e. public, self, associative and structural. In relation to fathers with mental health problems, these types may be described as follows:

→ **Public stigma:** occurs when negative reactions and discriminatory behaviours are directed to people who are perceived to have a stigmatising condition. Fathers with mental health problems often feel judged for their (perceived or actual) inability to meet the traditional paternal responsibilities of provider, protector and role-model. Such judgements can come from both service providers and other parents. Many fathers feel that because of their illness they are automatically seen as a risk to their children, and so are 'under observation'. Similarly, some express the concern that if they access services, or reveal the true extent of their problems to service providers, they will be at risk of losing child custody.

→ **Self-stigma:** involves stigmatised individuals internalising the stereotypes and discriminatory narratives that are directed towards them. Whether it is true or not, some fathers internalise the view that because of their mental illness they will find it difficult or impossible to be a 'good enough parent'. Some fathers with mental health problems feel that they have failed to perform the activities and fulfil fathering responsibilities, such as breadwinning and providing moral guidance. These feelings may exist in spite of emotional engagement and devotion to their children.

→ **Stigma by association:** occurs when stigma is directed towards those associated with a discredited individual. For fathers, this may involve their children or partners being teased, abused, blamed, pitied or avoided as a result of having a family member with mental health problems. Stigma by association may also negatively impact the communicative dynamics within families. For instance, some men hide their mental health problems from their families in an attempt to spare them from stigma by association.

→ **Structural stigma:** involves the perpetuation of stigma and discrimination by society's institutions, as present in jurisdictions where a parent's psychiatric disorder is a legally accepted reason for custody loss, as is the case in some states in the US (Kaplan et al, 2009). As discussed below, some fathers feel that their mental health is used against them when decisions are made regarding access and childcare.

These four types of stigma are further discussed in Price-Robertson et al, in press.

> **Practice reflections**
>
> 1. What beliefs do you hold regarding the parenting capacity of people with mental health problems?
> 2. Consider the last time you saw fathers' mental health represented in the media. Was it discussed within the context of violence? Were fathers' strengths and capacities considered?
> 3. Do you think it is possible that experiencing mental health problems could ultimately help some men become better fathers than they otherwise would have been?

Stigma and fathers' help-seeking behaviours

Price-Robertson et al, (in press) found that traditional masculine ideals may reinforce a sense of isolation for fathers, who are often reluctant to talk to their families and friends about their mental health problems. As one father in Reupert and Maybery's (2009) study said:

> 'Through this whole time my [now ex-] wife had friends to talk to because women support other women, but men don't... Men are supposed to be tough and strong... As a kid, I was taught by my brother to take pain and bear it, so that's what I did.' (p65)

Indeed, some fathers completely hide their mental health problems from their families. In one case outlined by Galasinski (2013), a 72-year-old father, with diagnosed bipolar disorder for over 40 years, had never told his wife and children about his disorder.

Many fathers with mental health problems do not engage with health and welfare services (Featherstone, 2009; Maxwell et al, 2012). In general, men are less likely than women to seek professional help for a range of problems, including mental health concerns, physical illness and disability, and stressful life events (Addis & Mahalik, 2003; Galdas et al 2005). This reluctance to access services is the same for fathers, who *'are much less likely than mothers to seek out health workers, community welfare professionals and parents' groups if they need support in their role as carer'* (Berlyn et al, 2008 p5).

Stigma plays a critical role in shaping men's health behaviours. Men who fall short of masculine ideals are more likely to be the subject of stigmatisation (Price-Robertson, 2015). For example, in many cultures, men with infertility problems are stigmatised for their perceived deficiencies in virility and potency (Inhorn, 2004). Mental health problems, too, may expose men to situations and experiences that are starkly at odds with the traditional masculine ideals of self-reliance, physical toughness and emotional control (Galasinski, 2013). Moreover, mental health problems may undermine men's ability to meet the expectations of fatherhood, such as breadwinning. In this regard, Galasinski (2013) recently wrote of the *'inherent contradiction between the dominant expectations of fatherhood and the dominant discourses and imagery of mental illness'* (p1). Alongside the more general threat of mental illness stigma, fathers with mental health problems also face the prospect of being discriminated against for their loss of masculine and paternal status. In the face of such a threat, it is little wonder that fathers can be reluctant to share their struggles with others.

> **Practice reflections**
>
> 1. To what extent do you think fathers are still judged according to their capacity to provide for their families? Does this differ according to ethnicity, class and geography?
> 2. What do you think are the main reasons that men are more reluctant than women to seek help for their problems?

Stigma towards fathers in the health and welfare sector

Unfortunately, even when fathers do come into contact with health or welfare service systems, they may be met by judgement and discrimination. Whether their perception is accurate or not, it is common for fathers to believe that service providers ignore their needs or are biased against them (Price-Robertson et al, in press). Stigma experienced by fathers with mental health problems is particularly salient in the child welfare sector. Many fathers (and mothers) fear losing custody of their children. Many believe the welfare system overemphasises their psychopathology and is preoccupied with parental deficits and risks (Reupert et al, 2012). In particular, fathers *'strongly believed their mental illness was a significant negative factor when decisions were being made regarding access'* and that their illness had been used against them in childcare disputes (Reupert & Maybery, 2009, p64). As one father noted:

> 'Mental illness is a powerful thing to use… In custody cases, it is an easy thing for people to use … more negative than if [you] bash your wife, and kids, or [if you are] drunk all the time or stoned.' (Reupert & Maybery, 2009, p64)

While it is important to emphasise that these are individual fathers' perceptions and are not necessarily indicative of the actual presence of stigma, there is reason to believe that some fathers do encounter both structural and public stigma in the child welfare system. Studies in Australia (Berlyn et al, 2008; Russell et al, 1999) and the UK (Featherstone, 2009; Scourfield, 2003; 2006a) found that negative or ambivalent attitudes towards fathers are common in child welfare settings. For instance, in an analysis of the child protection system in the UK, Scourfield (2003; 2006a) identified two dominant discourses towards male clients: they were seen as 'a threat', presumed to be violent and coercive; and, as being of 'no use', said to *'spend little time on, and have few skills for, either child care or domestic work'* (Scourfield, 2006a, p81). It is unsurprising, then, that in Featherstone's study (2009) exploring the experiences of fathers whose children were involved in social care services in the UK, participants tended to be very critical of social workers, routinely describing them as *'on the woman's side'* (p163).

Prejudice against fathers in welfare settings is thought to be related to the female-dominated workforce, the traditional societal assumption that child-rearing is predominantly a woman's responsibility, and workers' fears of violent male clients (Featherstone, 2009; Maxwell et al, 2012). While a bias against fathers is clearly problematic, it is important to acknowledge that this is a complex area of scholarship and practice, and that workers' assumptions and fears often stem from very real issues: family violence perpetrated by fathers is a feature of many child protection cases (Featherstone, 2009), and, in at least some cases, *'fathers involvement with their children can be linked to their desire to retain control and further undermine women'* (Featherstone, 2009, p171). Nonetheless, while some men with a mental health problem do pose a risk to their families, this is certainly not the case for all of such fathers (Reupert & Maybery, 2009). Indeed, public perceptions of those with mental health problems as criminally dangerous appear to be greatly exaggerated (Stuart & Arboldea-Flòrez, 2001).

Practice reflections

1. Are negative or ambivalent attitudes towards fathers present in your organisation?
2. If your work involves contact with men who are violent or manipulative, what measures could you take to ensure that this contact does not colour your views of all male clients?
3. What factors help you judge whether a male client may be a threat to you or someone else? To what extent does his mental health status inform your judgement?

Challenging stigma

While it is important that anti-stigma strategies are evidence based, there is a paucity of research in this area, especially in relation to fathers with mental health problems. This section provides an overview of the different approaches that may be used, and how these might relate to fathers.

Public attitudes

Education – including but not limited to awareness campaigns, podcasts, advisements, video and movies – is a common strategy that aims to shift public attitudes toward those with a mental health problems. In relation to fathers, education might counter stereotypes that such men are dangerous or otherwise incapable of caring for children. More broadly, outdated or patronising representations of fathers (e.g. fathers as 'part time parents', 'baby entertainers' or 'Mr Mum' (Petroski & Edley, 2006)) need to be resisted and reframed, so that fathers are seen in terms of the unique and varied contributions they bring to family life. The public is also educated about mental health via the media, albeit in often sensational and inaccurate ways. News and entertainment representations tend to emphasise the violent, delusional and irrational behaviour of those with mental health problems (Stuart, 2006). Education is most effective when it is multi-faceted and includes confronting common myths (e.g. dangerousness), is targeted and audience specific (e.g. police, welfare workers), and includes the voices of consumers (Queensland Alliance for Mental Health, 2010).

Emerging evidence demonstrates that positive contact with someone with mental health problems is effective in increasing empathy and understanding (Gordon, 2005). Given the high prevalence of mental health problems in the community (i.e. one in five people affected in any given year (Australian Bureau of Statistics, 2008)), it is reasonable to suggest that many people are already in contact with someone with a mental health problems. The problem is that many do not disclose their mental health status for fear of judgement and discrimination. Indirect contact, through sports role models or other public figures discussing their mental health might promote acceptance, as long as the social distance is not too large and the public is able to identify with the individual (Queensland Alliance for Mental Health, 2010). Contact is effective when it involves debunking myths associated with mental health problems (e.g. that men with a mental illness are always a danger to their children), when there is opportunity for discussion, and where it occurs within the context of a pre-existing relationship (e.g. with a co-worker or neighbour) (Queensland Alliance for Mental Health, 2010).

Professional attitudes

Research has repeatedly demonstrated that different professional groups hold stigmatising views towards those with a mental illness (Reupert & Maybey, in press). Some professional groups appear to hold more stigmatising attitudes than others, with one study finding that psychiatrists rated persons with mental illness as more dangerous, less skilled and more socially disturbing than did psychologists, nurses or other therapists (Lauber et al, 2006). Such a finding suggests that different anti-stigma approaches are required for different groups. While efforts at educating medical practitioners about father-inclusive practice are promising (e.g. Fletcher et al, 2012), it is unclear what impact they may have made. Comparatively little attention has been dedicated to changing the negative or ambivalent attitudes towards fathers that have been identified in social work and child welfare environments, despite repeated calls (e.g. Maxwell et al, 2012). Increasing the number of male workers is a common suggestion for achieving such attitudinal changes (Berlyn et al, 2008), though attracting male workers to such positions has proven difficult (Featherstone, 2009).

Fathers' internalised stigma

Self-empowerment is at the core of changing men's negative views of themselves as fathers. While insight tends to be regarded as advantageous for treatment, it may also be accompanied by internalised negative stereotypes about mental health problems (e.g. 'I'm a bad parent because I have a mental illness') (Reupert & Maybery, in press). This means that clinicians need to carefully balance the promotion of insight with feelings of competence so that fathers might find new and adaptive ways of thinking about themselves. Promoting positive self-talk might be incorporated within cognitive behaviour therapy (e.g. 'Just because I have a mental illness, doesn't mean I can't be a good father'). Men's self-help groups might also provide a useful source of support and a safe environment in which to discuss their experience of fathering and mental illness.

Practice reflections

1. What might your role be in shifting negative attitudes towards fathers with mental health problems? Could you contribute to efforts at anti-stigma education? Are there ways to challenge discriminatory attitudes within your organisation?

2. Think about fathers you have worked with. Have you noticed any practices or interventions that have contributed to their feelings of self-worth and empowerment?

Promoting father-inclusive practice

While it is important to challenge attitudes, practices and policies that stigmatise fathers, more is needed. The absence of stigma does not automatically ensure that services will be responsive to fathers. Another, more active step is required: health and child welfare services must become father-inclusive. Being father-inclusive does not mean that the very real risks of male-perpetrated family violence are minimised or ignored. Rather, it involves services acknowledging that fathers matter, and making efforts towards ensuring that fathers become part of the solution to family problems. Specific to child welfare, Scourfield (2006b, p446) argues that workers need to *'see men as both risk and resource for women and children'*, and actively work to engage men in assessments and family interventions.

Berlyn et al (2008) found that *'programs for men have a tendency to be a sideline operation to main service activities'*, and that the services that were most effective at attracting fathers had *'made an organisation-wide commitment to increasing father participation, providing staff with training on engaging fathers, and creating staff positions dedicated to involving fathers in the service's activities'* (p5). Maxwell et al (2012) echoed this finding in their recent review of the factors that have been found to facilitate father engagement with services. Such factors included:

→ **Early identification and involvement:** where fathers are invited to engage with services as early as possible. While it is often most effective to engage with fathers in hospital at the time of their child's birth, many young or disadvantaged fathers are excluded at this time. Health professionals might encourage fathers to attend appointments related to pregnancy and then later for meetings related to child care. Similarly, antenatal classes should include information specifically for fathers.

→ **A proactive approach to engaging fathers:** which involves practices such as visiting fathers at home, ensuring that services' opening hours accommodate working fathers, displaying positive images of fathers and their children, employing male staff, and advertising in locations such as sports centres and workplaces.

→ **Making services relevant to fathers:** by focusing on their self-identified needs and offering services in formats that appeal to them. Even when multiple risk factors exist in fathers' lives, many men do not perceive a need for parenting support. Rather, they tend to be most concerned with issues of employment, substance abuse and mental health. When they do access family services, many men prefer outdoor activities with their children and skill-based education, as opposed to class-room style parenting education or discussion groups.

Practice reflections

1. What does your organisation currently do to promote the engagement and involvement of fathers? What more could be done?

2. Are you missing important opportunities to engage with fathers in the first stages of working with families?

3. How could your organisation's current services be modified to be made more relevant to fathers?

Conclusion

While a common experience for both mothers and fathers, it is likely that mental illness stigma, at least in part, manifests along gendered lines. Thus, it is important to understand how stigma can influence the lives of fathers with mental health problems. The limited research on this topic suggests that mental illness stigma can have an impact on the way fathers participate in family life, how they see themselves as fathers, their help-seeking behaviours, and how they are treated by health and welfare professionals.

There is no magic bullet when it comes to preventing mental health stigma directed towards parents. Such stigma manifests in numerous domains: from public attitudes about parenting, to professional attitudes and behaviours, to men's own feelings about themselves and their capacity to provide care. It is likely that efforts at prevention will need to focus on each of these domains. More research is required to better understand how the community and different professional groups perceive and behave towards fathers with mental health problems, and how to most effectively change attitudes and practices that see vulnerable fathers and their families subject to stigmatisation.

References

Addis M & Mahalik J (2003) Men, masculinity, and the contexts of help seeking. *American Psychologist* **58** (1) 5–14.

Australian Bureau of Statistics (2008) *National Survey of Mental Health and Wellbeing: Summary of results, 2007* [online]. Canberra: ABS. Available at: http://www.abs.gov.au/AUSSTATS/abs@.nsf/DetailsPage/4326.02007?OpenDocument (accessed September 2015).

Berlyn C, Wise S & Soriano G (2008) *Engaging Fathers in Child and Family Services: Participation, perceptions and good practice* [online]. Canberra: National Evaluation Consortium. Available at: https://www.dss.gov.au/our-responsibilities/families-and-children/publications-articles/number-22-engaging-fathers-in-child-and-family-services-participation-perceptions-and-good-practice (accessed September 2015).

Elgar F, Mills R, McGrath P, Waschbusch D & Brownridge D (2007) Maternal and paternal depressive symptoms and child maladjustment: the mediating role of parental behavior. *Journal of Abnormal Child Psychology* **35** (6) 943–955.

Featherstone B (2009) *Contemporary Fathering: Theory, policy and practice.* Bristol: The Policy Press.

Fletcher R, Maharaj ON, Fletcher Watson CH, May C, Skeates N & Gruenert S (2012) Fathers with mental illness: implications for clinicians and health services. *MJA Open* **1** 34-36.

Galasinski D (2013) *Fathers, Fatherhood and Mental Illness: A discourse analysis of rejection.* Hampshire, UK: Palgrave Macmillan.

Galdas P, Cheater F & Marshall P (2005) Men and health help-seeking behaviour: literature review. *Journal of Advanced Nursing* **49** (6) 616–623.

Gordon S (2005) *The Power of Contact.* Wellington: Case Consulting.

Hinshaw S (2005) The stigmatization of mental illness in children and parents: developmental issues, family concerns, and research needs. *Journal of Child Psychology and Psychiatry and Allied Disciplines* **46** (7) 714–734.

Inhorn M (2004) Middle Eastern masculinities in the age of new reproductive technologies: male infertility and stigma in Egypt and Lebanon. *Medical Anthropology Quarterly* **18** (2) 162–182.

Kaplan K, Kottsieper P, Scott J, Salzer M & Solomon P (2009) Adoption and Safe Families Act State Statutes regarding parental mental illnesses: a review and targeted intervention. *Psychiatric Rehabilitation Journal* **33** (2) 91–94.

Lauber C, Nordt C, Braunschweig C & Rössler W (2006) Do mental health professionals stigmatize their patients? *Acta Psychiatra Scandinavia* **113** 51–59.

Maxwell N, Scourfield J, Featherstone B, Holland S & Tolman R (2012) Engaging fathers in child welfare services: a narrative review of recent research evidence. *Child and Family Social Work* **17** (2) 160–169.

Petroski D & Edley P (2006) Stay-at-home fathers: masculinity, family, work and gender. *The Electronic Journal of Communication* **16** (3-4).

Phelan J (2005) Geneticization of deviant behaviour and consequences of stigma: the case of mental illness. *Journal of Health and Social Behavior* **46** (4) 307–322.

Price-Robertson R (2015) *Fatherhood and Mental Illness: A review of key issues (CFCA Paper No. 30)* [online]. Melbourne: Australian Institute of Family Studies. Available at: https://aifs.gov.au/cfca/publications/fatherhood-and-mental-illness (accessed September 2015).

Price-Robertson R, Reupert A & Maybery D (in press) Fathers' experiences of mental illness stigma: scoping review and implications for prevention. *Advances in Mental Health.*

Pryor J & Reeder G (2011) HIV-related stigma. In: J Hall, B Hall & C Cockerell (Eds) *HIV/AIDS in the Post-HAART Era: Manifestations, treatment, and epidemiology* pp 790-806. Shelton, CT: PMPH-USA.

Queensland Alliance for Mental Health (2010) *From Discrimination to Social Inclusion. A review of the literature on anti-stigma initiatives in mental health* [online]. Available at: http://www.mhct.org/documents/Lit_review_proof_140410.pdf (accessed September 2015).

Reupert A & Maybery D (2009) Fathers' experience of parenting with a mental illness. *Families in Society: The Journal of Contemporary Social Sciences* **90** (1) 61–68.

Reupert A & Maybery D (in press) Stigma in families where a parent has a mental illness. In: A Reupert, D Maybery, J Nicholson, M Göpfert & M Seeman (Eds) (3rd edition). *Parental Psychiatric Disorder: Distressed parents and their families*. London: Cambridge Univeristy Press.

Reupert A, Maybery D & Kowalenko N (2012) Children whose parents have a mental illness: prevalence, need and treatment. *Medical Journal of Australia* **16** 7–9.

Russell G, Barclay L, Edgecombe G, Donovan J, Habib G & Callaghan H (1999) *Fitting Fathers into Families: Men and the fatherhood role in contemporary Australia.* Canberra: Department of Family and Community Services.

Scourfield J (2003) *Gender and Child Protection.* Basingstoke and London: Palgrave Macmillan.

Scourfield J (2006a) Gendered organizational culture in child protection social work. *Social Work* **51** (1) 80–82.

Scourfield J (2006b). The challenge of engaging fathers in the child protection process. *Critical Social Policy* **26** (2) 440–449.

Stuart H (2006) Media portrayal of mental illness and its treatment. What effect does it have on people with mental illness? *CNS Drugs* **20** (2) 90–106.

Stuart H & Arboleda-Flòrez J (2001) A public health perspective on violent offenses among persons with mental illness. *Psychiatric Services* **52** (5) 654–659.

Conceptual models

Chapter 14

Learning from success: conceptual introduction

By Professor Shula Ramon

Failure and success in working with people who use mental health and child care services are key points on a continuum of intervention outcomes and processes. These are relative terms by definition, as they are measured by their proximity to a desired outcome. Furthermore, as there are at least two stakeholders in an encounter between professionals and people using health and social care services, it is likely that what is defined as either success or failure would vary between them, though they may agree as to what will constitute major failure or success.

Failure is usually defined as lack of success in achieving a desired outcome, and most people prefer not to talk about it. This reluctance to look at failure comes out of its negative connotations for the personal and professional standing of those involved, even when the circumstances may be the core reason for it. The prevention of failure may become a shared objective between a service provider and a service user, but would be unlikely to be presented as such, given the formal emphasis on success in most care services.

Usually, success is willingly spoken about, even paraded and celebrated, because it marks the opposite of failure, namely the accomplishment of achieving the desired outcome, often motivating the actors to strive for further success and to set the bar higher than before.

Occasions on which this is not the case occur in care practice, and in any other service practice, when it is tacitly assumed that the specific success is unlikely to be maintained and is perceived as only short lived, often not celebrated. For example, in a small scale study of how people moved from a psychiatric hospital admission to the community (Ramon, 1991) most of the participants mentioned no ceremony to celebrate success upon leaving, often being encouraged just to take their belongings in a plastic bag and leave the ward via a back door, with no one waiting for them in the community to celebrate their achievement. The very term 'discharge', used to denote leaving a hospital ward, suggests a military order rather than the completion of a therapeutic interaction.

Yet the entry to a psychiatric hospitalisation episode is marked by a 'degradation ceremony', a term coined by Garfinkel (1956) in describing the meaning of the process of re-configuring one's past history in the light of the failure that such an entry signifies. This type of failure is all too often portrayed as an individual failure, rather than a possible system failure. Only rarely are providers called to account for an admission, even though an admission is perceived as a failure, often looked upon as an inevitable one. The belief in the inevitability of an admission is a way of justifying chronicity and the belief that the person has no future prospects of improvement in their mental health state. Only rarely do we come across a ceremony of re-gradation, in which the success of recovery from a mental health crisis of a person, or a whole group, a transition from an institution to the community, is noted (e.g. Trieste opening of the hospital to artists and to the community at large – see Del Guidice et al, 1990).

Turning a psychiatric hospital admission into a success can be an integral part of the process of recovery in its new meaning, as highlighted by Patricia Deegan, who describes her ability to decide and plan such an admission as evidence of being in control (Deegan, 1997).

The tradition of learning from failure

Learning theories have taught us that we learn best from success, rather than from failure (Schon, 1991). Experiments have highlighted that success leads to a re-validation of our abilities and aspirations, and to an increase in self confidence, motivating us to re-invest in new learning.

Failure, meanwhile, makes us doubt our abilities, weakens our motivation to invest in new learning, and may lead to reduced aspirations and self-esteem, as well as moving away from a particular avenue of self-investment altogether. Because failure is frowned upon in most societies, but especially in modern ones, we tend to engage in strategies of hiding it, including hiding it from ourselves. At times, given guidance and support without condemnation, we are able to reflect and analyse failure, as well as engage in learning how to prevent it from happening. However, on the whole the training of all helping professions does not include learning from success as a strategy, beyond following a list of actions proven by past experience to lead to success.

Given the intensity of focus on success and competition in wider society as a major criterion of the value of an individual, a collective, a company and a system, it is a strange paradox that we are not engaging systematically in learning from success within the helping professions, either in pre-qualifying training or afterwards. There is no simple or straightforward answer to this paradox – it is usually not even raised. Perhaps the fact that the helping professions do not focus on economic success, which is the one that counts most in the modern world, leads to the de-valuing of any other success.

The competitive nature of success in wider society may be another component that makes helping professions recoil from focusing on success, as this type of competition has no ethical place within the range of activities these professions engage in. It could also be that the often observed partial success is perceived as not good enough.

Furthermore, within the helping professions the partial answer is the reliance on caution in focusing on failure as the dominant feature of our practice, given the complexity of the issues we are dealing with, as well as the focus on risk avoidance. Thus, not focusing on success is a way of accepting lower expectations of both clients and providers, which can be more easily achieved. Success as a result of professional activities within the field of mental health has all too often been related to making people more comfortable, reducing suffering, reducing negative risk and increasing conformity with social norms, accepting mental ill health as something we cannot change and need to accept as a given. Indeed, traditional psychiatric textbooks teach us to judge patients by the degree to which they accept their illness as a sign of insight, to view their non-patienthood ambitions as untenable, and to require of them to give these ambitions up altogether (Lysaker *et al*, 2007).

Although we work and live today with a much wider range of views on the potential of people experiencing mental ill health than before, some of which will be looked at later, recent research carried out for the Time-to-Change five years anti-stigma project has found that mental health service providers had a more pessimistic view of this group's potential than the general public (Brindle, 2013). This may be explained by the fact that they encounter more of the difficulties and failures experienced than the public does, but equally they are likely to see more of the successes, yet seem to remain focused on the failures.

Concentrating on failure is closely connected to avoiding risks in a culture that fosters fear of risk taking and back covering to prevent being blamed when things go wrong. Paradoxically, it is also a culture that celebrates risk taking when successful, in business, arts and in sport. While the wish to avoid harm to self and to others is understandable and desirable, each of us – lay people, service providers or service users and carers – knows that calculated risk taking is a necessary ingredient of living and of moving from one stage of life to another. This common sense knowledge is corroborated by research evidence of human development (Erickson, 1968), yet denied when it comes to the field of mental health and illness. Politicians and mass media also take prominent roles in blaming either providers and/or service users when things go wrong, as do service managers, thus participating in promoting a 'blame culture' that mitigates against taking positive, calculated risks. In the various training courses available, service providers are often given detailed instructions as to what they need to do to avoid risk taking, but much less attention (if any) is paid to how to set up calculated, desired activities that contain some risk. They therefore ignore existing knowledge that we perform better in tasks we wish to undertake, than those dictated to us by others.

Marie Diggins' chapter (Chapter 15) explains in detail what success is in parental mental health and child care, highlighting that the definition of success, its instances and magnitude, differ among the key stakeholders, be they parents, children, young carers, child care and mental health providers. Not surprisingly, the differences relate to the vested interests each stakeholder has, but also to their subjective and intersubjective experience, as well as to their order of priorities. The bar set by professionals for specific success is often higher in scope than the one identified by parents and children, raising the possibility of a mismatch of expectations which may contribute to a lower level of success. Moreover, both parents and children are able to identify success of intervention processes and not only of outcomes, as the processes focus on the relational aspect of the intervention which is often not perceived as part of the outcome.

Writing on safeguarding children, both Marie Diggins and Andy Quin (see Chapter 16) highlight that parents were more at ease in identifying success than the providers, and were able to identify the role of service providers in this achievement, as well as their own contribution. The providers' difficulty in apportioning success to a parent whose child has been taken away highlights the frustration felt by the provider at the partial failure of the parent, and the barrier of recognising partial success by such a parent. This is an issue deserving our attention, not only because it may confirm the fear that failure may be lurking even when success is taking place, but also perhaps because it illustrates providers' scepticism that the parents' effort – and their own effort – is not going to be sufficient to ensure success. Andy Quin's observation that children safeguarding boards were not interested in the voices of the parents or the children indicates another key issue – that of the aspirations of the managerial and political partners of achieving safeguarding through meeting administrative objectives of a goal which is primarily not administrative, but relational in essence. This lack of interest in the views of these two key stakeholders does not bode well for the success of the safeguarding system as a whole, while confirming its focus on preventing and reducing failure instead.

What would it mean to learn systematically from success?

Such learning would include mapping the processes leading to a particular successful outcome, as well as the facilitators and barriers of success and analysing the intersectionality of such a map. Looking at the degree of shared decision making in deciding on a specific outcome and on the process of achieving it would be another layer of learning. Understanding the micro, mezzo and macro levels at which the outcome is primarily located alongside the facilitators and barriers is another central angle of learning.

Learning by example has been found to be a particularly suitable way to introduce desirable change (Rosenfeld *et al*, 2010; Ramon, 2011) which requires unlearning and re-learning by providers and service users alike. Motivational interviewing (Miller & Rollnick, 2012) offers another route for clients, which focuses on eliciting the value of a specific change to achieving the aims a person has, alongside boosting confidence in their capacities. Group learning is another methodological device that can help enable a group to reflect on how to achieve objectives which, from a traditional perspective on mental health, seem unachievable, but become achievable after shifting our perceptions of what a person with a disability can achieve (Rapp & Goscha, 2012).

A fascinating example of research on the meaning of success in domestic violence perpetrators programmes (Westmarland & Kelly, 2013) illustrates the scope and depth of success for women victims of such violence, their children, and the perpetrators. Based on interviews of all stakeholders (perpetrators, women victims, providers and commissioners), they highlight that the substance of success in such programmes is much wider than the formal definition of success. Success includes factors such as improved couple relationships underpinned by respect and effective communication, expanded space for action, empowering through restoring their voice and ability to make choices while improving well-being, safe, positive and shared parenthood, men's enhanced awareness of self and others, and a safer, healthier childhood for their children.

The conceptual underpinnings of learning from success in health and social care

The strengths approach

Adherents of the strengths approach believe that people who use health and social care services have strengths and not only weaknesses (Rapp & Goscha, 2012). Furthermore, the strengths may be there only potentially and need to be developed by service users with support from providers. Such a belief relates closely to the underlying assumption that service users are people rather than a collection of disabilities, and by virtue of being human are likely to have abilities as well as weaknesses (Ryan & Deci, 2001). These abilities may not have been developed to their full potential either because of the limitations imposed by a disability or by the social and professional perspectives which view them as incapable of anything. The latter is a reflection of the impact of the master status of being a person with a disability, in which we name the person by their disability or diagnosis (e.g. 'schizophrenic' rather than s/he is a person to whom having schizophrenia has been attributed, 'paraplegic' 'blind') and literally forget about any other quality they possess (Goffman, 1963).

The strengths approach follows in principle the social model of disability (Swain *et al*, 2004), which argues that people with disabilities are people first, with many qualities, and that many of the restrictions on their abilities and contribution to society are due to social barriers, rather than the implications of the specific disability they may have. The achievements of people with disabilities, especially physical disabilities, exemplified in the 2012 London Paralympic Games and the removal of a number of physical barriers to physical mobility which led to their increased visibility, evidences the value of the social model of disability. Coming originally from Aristotle's focus on human flourishing (Ryan & Deci, 2012), but developed within the helping disciplines initially in social work (Saleebey, 1992), the strengths approach focuses on the why and how of developing disabled people's strengths, instead of dwelling only on their disability. The justification for this approach is closely related to the focus on success, where the development of strengths comes to compensate for the weaknesses caused by the disability, as well as to develop a more balanced life. Furthermore, the development of potential strengths leads to a growing capacity and motivation to undertake new tasks, as there is nothing like success to lead to further success. Rapp & Goscha (2012), who have extensively developed this approach in the context of mental health work, highlight the importance of working with providers teams and community networks to develop readiness to embrace the strengths approach and to acquire the skills for this type of work. Their work has also led to the beginning of evaluation research on the value of this approach (Fukai *et al*, 2012, Teague *et al*, 2012).

Unlike the Capabilities Approach (Nussbaum, 2001) which looks at the gap between functionality (people as they are) and capability (their potential) from a philosophical and social structural perspective, or unlike the social model of disability, the strengths approach does not include an analysis of the structural layer.

The new meaning of recovery

The new meaning of recovery in mental health focuses on the ability to live better with the illness and to live beyond it (Davidson, 2003), as well as on moving away from the traditional medical model focus on symptoms reduction and repression in favour of a more psychosocial approach. In particular, recovery aims to enable a unique individual journey in which the person finds what is meaningful to them, including reconnection to other people, groups and communities (Bird *et al*, 2014). Side by side with the individual focus, this approach also entails an emphasis on stigma reduction and the acknowledgement of social structural barriers to recovery (Tew *et al*, 2012). It has taken from the strengths approach the belief that people experiencing mental ill health have a lot to offer to themselves and to others, exemplified by the construction of the recovery colleges and peer support workers (Meddings *et al*, 2015), and a variety of service user-led projects, as well as by the creative contributions of many individuals who have psychiatric labels (Longden, 2010). This approach recognises that providers, politicians and the general public need to learn from the experiential knowledge of people who use mental health services, who should also be partners to policy and intervention decisions, as well as to research about recovery. This aspect challenges the belief in the supremacy of scientific knowledge as the only valid type of knowledge, to which many professionals adhere, even though the lack of good enough knowledge of a number of mental health areas is patent, or contested for good reasons.

The recovery approach is criticised for encouraging people to take on the responsibility for their lives, alongside giving them more control over their lives which is interpreted as allegiance to neoliberalism (Harper & Speed, 2012), and as a devaluation of madness (Beresford, 2015). Outside of the realm of mental ill health, control over one's life is a desirable aim, one that does indeed carry greater responsibility with it than when one does not aim to be in such control. This is a universal value which predates neoliberalism, and is more closely related to the enlightenment ideals. In the recovery approach, success is not measured in financial terms, but in the development of one's agency, meaningful activities and abilities in any aspect of living, especially in giving to other people in a variety of ways, in becoming more connected to others, and in looking after one's well-being better. The pressure to take responsibility for oneself is interpreted in this critique as an attempt by society to stop its obligations towards people who are experiencing mental ill health, which is indeed a feature of neoliberalism, but is not one the promoters of the new meaning of recovery adhere to at all.

The recovery approach does pay considerable attention to knowledge coming from experts in experience, and upholds individuals in mental distress the right to support and to their own individual journey of recovery, but does not romanticise madness as more valued than other life experiences. On the whole, the recovery approach too pays scant attention to the social structural dimension, apart from its foci on stigma and on social inclusion.

Agency, empowerment, reciprocity and collaboration

Historically, the concept of success came to Western culture from Calvinism in the 17th century, where it was viewed as evidence that the person is doing the right thing by God. Its cultural connotations in the 21st century are located more with financial success, the capitalist system, neoliberalism and individualism. It also resonates with artistic and sport achievements, which call for a high level of risk taking and of tolerating uncertainty. The latter focuses on the role of agency (Archer, 2003), yet the components of empowerment, reciprocity and collaboration in the context of both economic and non-economic success should not be under estimated. Agency is that abstract yet specific, sense of self. Breakwell (1986), coming from a social psychological perspective, investigated the issue of people with a threatened identity due to the impact of a variety of adverse events in their lives, such as becoming unemployed, going through a mental health crisis, being a black person in a racist society, or being abused. Having such an uncertain identity calls for the development of specific coping mechanisms, which may vary from a constructive re-evaluation, sense of loss of part – or the whole – of the self, attempting to assume a more desirable identity ('passing'), and seeking power and autonomy. These examples highlight the impact of structure on agency and vice versa.

Empowerment is a complex concept, as only the person can empower themselves, yet evidence highlights the crucial element of the need to know that someone else believes in them as a facilitator of empowerment and the positive belief in oneself (Glover, 2012). Often empowerment translates as being given support and opportunities in which to develop strengths and to fulfil ambitions, the belief in the whole person rather than in the stigmatised persona, the readiness to take the risk of taking responsibility, and the participation in shared decision making. The example of peer support workers practised in Australia, Canada, Israel, New Zealand, the UK and US illustrates the duality of existing as a person who uses mental health services yet is also able to make a significant contribution to the lives of others with mental health difficulties, alongside professional providers. It highlights not only the ability to exercise agency and empowerment, but also reciprocity and collaboration among people who formally do not have equal power to service providers. A considerable shift in the beliefs of providers had to take place for this to happen, towards accepting the strengths of this group, the value of their experiential knowledge, their empathy capacity, their readiness to learn, and their readiness to take a high level of risk of moving from what has been allocated to them as their traditional comfort zone (Ashcraft & Anthony, 2005; Repper & Carter, 2011; Shears & Ramon, 2012). Likewise, the involvement of citizens using mental health services as co-researchers or as user-led researchers signifies the change in valuing the knowledge they bring with them as necessary within mental health research, a type of knowledge that improves the quality of this research, while enabling them to acquire new skills, and for some a new career path (Ramon, 2003)

A note on intersectionality

The conceptual map of learning from success outlined above remains incomplete if we do not take into account the intersectional interaction between the large number of the factors mentioned above (Hanishevsky, 2012, Yuval-Davis, 2011), or the combined impact of these inter-relationships. All too often we pay no more than lip service to the impact of factors such as ethnicity, gender, poverty, power (Kaminskiy, 2015) and organisational structure (Ramon, 2011), because these are treated as background variables which can be put aside. However, both conceptually and in everyday living, they do matter objectively in terms of life circumstances, and subjectively in terms of the way we perceive our place in the world and that of others. These factors impact on our agency, recognition by others (Fraser & Honneth, 2003), likelihood to be offered opportunities, ability to make use of opportunities and the development of resilience strategies against adversity. Consequently, they impact directly on the likelihood of achieving success.

Learning points

If success is to be taken seriously in connection with parental mental health and child care, than the following steps need to follow:

1. Success should be identified as an objective from the outset of an intervention.
2. Success should be celebrated when it takes place.
3. Training to recognise the value of success, its conceptual and values underpinning, the process of enabling it to happen and its facilitators and barriers is needed. Such training should be delivered not only to service providers, but also to service users and carers.
4. Positive, calculated, risk taking needs to be emphasised, and training to achieve it could be included in the training for success.
5. The relational aspect, the place of experiential knowledge, and the structural dimension of working with people experiencing mental ill health require not only acknowledgement, but to be much more centred upon in interventions with this client group.

References

Archer MS (2003) *Structure, Agency and the Internal Conversation*. Cambridge: Cambridge University Press.

Ashcraft L & Anthony W (2005) A story of transformation: an agency fully embraces recovery. *Behavioural Health Care Tomorrow* **14** 12–22.

Beresford P (2015) From 'recovery' to reclaiming madness. *Clinical Psychology Forum* **268** 16–20.

Breakwell GM (1986) *Threatened Identities*. London: Methuen.

Bird V, Leamy M, Tew J, Le Boutillier C, Williams J & Slade M (2014) Fit for purpose? Validation of a conceptual framework for personal recovery with current mental health consumers. *Australian & New Zealand Journal of Psychiatry* **48** (7) 644–653.

Boveink W (2012) Tree: towards recovery, empowerment and experiential expertise of users of psychiatric services. In: P Ryan, S Ramon & Greacen T (Eds) *Empowerment, Lifelong Learning and Recovery in Mental Health: Towards a new paradigm* (pp36-49). Basingstoke: Palgrave MacMillan.

Brindle D (2013) Mental health anti-stigma campaign fails to shift health professionals' attitudes. *The Guardian* 3 April.

Davidson L (2003) *Living Outside Mental Illness: Qualitative studies of recovery in schizophrenia.* New York: New York University Press.

Deegan PA (1997) Recovery and empowerment for people with psychiatric disabilities. *Social Work in Health Care* **25** (3) 11-24

Del Guidice G, Evaristo P & Reale M (1990) How can mental hospitals be phased out? In: S Ramon, MG Giannichedda (Ed.) *Psychiatry in Transition: The British and Italian Experiences* (pp199-207). London: Pluto Press.

Erickson EH (1968) *Identity, Youth and Crisis.* New York: Norton.

Fraser N & Honneth A (2003) *Redistribution or Recognition? A political-philosophical text.* London: Verso.

Fukai S, Goscha R, Rapp CA, Mabry A, Liddy P & Marty D (2012) Strengths model case management fidelity scores and clients outcomes. *Psychiatric Services* **63** (7) 708-710.

Garfinkel H (1956) Conditions of successful degradation ceremonies. *American Journal of Sociology* **61** 420-424.

Glover H (2012) Recovery, lifelong learning, empowerment and social inclusion – is a new paradigm emerging? In: P Ryan, S Ramon & T Greacen (Eds) *Empowerment, Lifelong Learning and Recovery in Mental Health: Towards a New Paradigm* (pp15-35) Basingstoke: Palgrave MacMillan.

Goffman I (1963) *Stigma: Notes on the Management of Spoiled Identities.* Englewood Cliffs: Prentice Hall.

Hanikvsky O (2012) Womens' health, men's health, gender and health: the implications of intersectionalities. *Social Science & Medicine* **74** (11) 1712–1772

Harper D & Speed E (2012) Uncovering recovery: the resistible rise of recovery and resilience. *Studies in Social Justice* **6** 9-26.

Kaminskiy E (2015) The elephant in the room: a theoretical examination of power for shared decision making in psychiatric medication management. *Intersectionalities: A Global Journal of Social Work Analysis, Research, Polity and Practice* **4** (2) 19-38.

Longden E (2010) Making sense of voices: a personal story of recovery. *Psychosis* **2** (3) 255-299.

Lysaker PH, Roe D & Yanos PT (2007) Toward understanding the insight paradox. *Schizophrenia Bulletin* **33** (1) 192-199.

Meddings S, Campbell E, Gugilietti S, Lambe H, Lock L, Byrne D & Whittington A (2015) From service user to students: the benefits of recovery colleges. In: D Harper and E Speed (Eds) *Clinical Psychology Forum* **268** Special issue on Recovery, 32-37.

Miller WR & Rolnick S (2012) *Motivational Interviewing.* London: Guildford Press.

Nussbaum M (2001) *Creating Capabilities: The human development.* Boston: Harvard University Press.

Ramon S (1991) The relevance of symbolic interaction perspectives to the conceptual and practice construction of leaving a psychiatric hospital. *Social Work & Social Sciences Review* **1** (3) 163-176.

Ramon S (2011) Organisational change in the context of recovery-oriented services. *Journal of Mental Health Workforce, Training, Education and Practice* **5** (1) 38-46.

Ramon S (Ed) (2003) *Users as Researchers in Health and Social Care: An Empowering Agenda?* Birmingham: Venture Press.

Rapp CA & Goscha RJ (2012) *The Strengths Model: A Recovery oriented Approach to Mental Health Services.* New York: Oxford University Press.

Repper J & Carter T (2011) A review of the literature on peer support in mental health. *Journal of Mental Health* **20** (4) 392-411.

Rosenfeld J, Gilat M & Tal D (2010) *Learning from Success in the Work of Youth Probation Officers.* Jerusalem: Myers-JDC-Brookdale Institute.

Ryan R & Deci E (2011) On happiness and human potentials: a review of research on hedonic and eudaimanic wellbeing. *Annual Review of Psychology* **52** 141-166.

Saleebey D (Ed.) (1992) *The Strengths Perspective in Social Work Practice.* New York: Longman.

Schon DA (1991) *The Reflective Turn: Case Studies for ND ON Educational Practice.* New York: Columbia University Teachers College.

Shears J & Ramon S (2012) Peer support workers: A critical analysis of an innovation in mental health. *Dialogue in Praxis* **1** (1-2) 71-87.

Swain J, French S, Barnes C & Thomas C (2004) *Disabling Barriers: Enabling Environments.* London: SAGE Publications.

Teague GB, Mueser KT & Rapp CA (2012) Advances in fidelity measures for mental health services. *Psychiatric Services* **63** (8) 765-771.

Tew J, Ramon S, Slade M, Bird V, Melton J & Le Boutillier C (2012) Social factors and recovery from mental health difficulties: a review of the evidence. *British Journal of Social Work* **42** 443-460.

Tudor K (1996) *Mental Health Promotion: Paradigms and Practice.* London: Routledge.

Westmarland N & Kelly L (2013) Why extending measurement of 'success' in domestic violence perpetrators programmes matters for social work. *British Journal of Social Work* **43** 1092-1110.

Yuval-Davis N (2011) *The Politics of Belonging: Intersectional Contestations.* London, UK: SAGE Publications.

Chapter 15

The added value of learning from success in parental mental health and child welfare work

By Dr Marie Diggins

Introduction

This article sets out the key findings from my PhD research in the form of an exploratory study of what constitutes success and the components and contributions that lead to success in parental mental health and child welfare work. The study was conducted between 2010 and 2012 in the London Borough of Lewisham and Liverpool. The report sets out the methodology and the methods used, followed by the main findings of the research and a discussion of their implications for practice. The limitations of the study are also considered and desirable future research is suggested.

The reasons for undertaking the study

Existing research has already established the potential direct and indirect impacts of mental illness on parenting, the parent/child relationship and the child, and the extent to which this poses a public health challenge (Rutter & Quinton, 1984; Kim-Cohen et al, 2003; Brandon, 2008; Cleaver et al, 2012). Problems with how adult and children's services understand and deliver support to parents with mental health problems and their children have also been identified. In contrast, there has been little research into how parents with mental health difficulties and their children can be supported successfully. 'What works', or what constitutes success in parental mental health and child welfare work is largely missing from the literature. The research aims to begin to address this gap by providing an original contribution to conceptualising and evaluating success in parental mental health and child welfare work.

The methodology and methods used

As an exploratory study, it covers a diverse population, i.e. different family members, different cultural and ethnic backgrounds, parents with different diagnoses, as well as statutory and voluntary sector agencies. Covering diversity is a key issue for this type of research in terms of exploring different opinions of success – both in outcomes and processes – rather than statistical representation of the population.

An interpretative approach was chosen for the study to enable the exploration of these issues. This was obtained by undertaking a multiple embedded case study methodology (Yin, 2003) with 12 families and their key workers from community mental health, children's social care and the voluntary sector. This methodology was chosen because it is suited to detailed, in-depth data collection involving multiple sources of information.

Data collection was undertaken in three incremental stages to ensure triangulation: individual interviews with parents, children and the professionals working with them; a review of the agency case files kept about the same families; and three focus groups (parents, children, mixed professionals). Participants were asked to identify successful situations that had occurred in each case study family during the 18 months before interview and give details about why these situations worked out well. The key messages arising from the analysis of the first two stages of data collection (interviews and case file reviews) were presented to each focus group to stimulate discussion and gain new inter-subjective insights into to the notion of success and the components leading to it. Thematic analysis was the method used for data analysis.

Given what is known about the over-representation of some Black and Minority Ethinic (BME) groups in mental health and statutory child care services, and the relationship between psychiatric disorders, various measures of poverty and the close links between deprivation and poor health, it was important that the study sites' populations offered the opportunity for identifying families that met these criteria. The two research sites and the organisations taking part were chosen in accordance with these aims.

Demographically, the populations in the two sites share similar characteristics (although Liverpool is much larger than Lewisham), such as a high degree of socio-economic deprivation, while the differences in context were not so large that they could not be reflected in the study.

Demographics of the sample

Forty nine individual interviews took place with parents, children and professionals (n=49), twenty two agency case files were reviewed (n=22) and three group discussions (n=3) were undertaken (one with parents, one with children and young people and one with a mixed group of professionals).

Mothers and fathers

Fathers are largely missing from the literature about parental mental health and child welfare and therefore it was important to try and gain the perspective of fathers. However this was not possible in practice, largely because of the very small number of fathers living with their children in this sample. Those that were did not meet the research criteria at the time of recruitment.

All of the parents in the 12 case studies were mothers (36 years to 50 years with a mean of 46 years). Nine of the mothers taking part are bringing up their children without support from the children's fathers. All of the mothers did not want the fathers of their children or their partners to be contacted about the research.

Children

There was an equal distribution of male and female children (45% male and 54% female), age ranging from nine years to 24 years, with a mean of 15 years. Eleven of the 12 children were young carers.

Family ethnicity

Recruiting a representative sample of families from BME communities was achieved. All three families recruited in the first research site were from BME communities. In the second research site, two of the nine families recruited came from BME communities and the remaining seven were all white British.

Socio-economic status

Eleven of the 12 families had two or more agencies supporting them at any one time during the two-year period before the research and six families had four or more agencies involved. These figures highlight the complexity of issues that can exist in families and how identifying and responding to complex needs can involve a significant number of agencies and resources.

All 12 families lived in local authority or housing association rented accommodation. All were living on low income and were in receipt of welfare benefits. All parents were unemployed and had been so for at least five years before interview. Recruiting families with these experiences makes it possible to explore the relationship between psychiatric disorders, various measures of poverty and the close links between deprivation and poor health.

Professionals

All of the mothers had contact with a CMHT professional (social worker, community psychiatric nurse or CMHT family support worker). All of the professionals interviewed from the voluntary sector organisations were qualified social workers and all but one had previous experience of working for a local authority in CSC. All of the case study families had had significant but episodic involvement with CSC social workers.

The main findings of the research

The starting point for this study was to identify successful situations in parental mental health and child welfare work. All of the case study families taking part had experienced 'success' (as defined by themselves) in one form or another in the 18–24 month period before the start of the research. Participants liked talking about success but said they rarely had the opportunity to do so and it was difficult for all participants to talk about what had worked out well without talking about the difficulties and barriers they experienced too. Voluntary sector professionals found talking about their own and their agency's contributions to positive family outcomes easier to identify and discuss than their statutory sector counterparts.

Success emerged as a dynamic state. For example, an improvement in the relationship between a parent and child may be the result of improved parental mental health facilitated by effective treatments, further facilitated by the commitment a parent and professional had made to their client-professional relationship. The same outcome for another family might have involved the need to overcome some barriers along the way, such as overcoming a parent's suspicion and fear about taking medication or having difficulty trusting a professional's recommendation based on previous negative experiences. In this case, further facilitation may be needed to overcome or negotiate these barriers before a final outcome is reached. A significant number of intermediary examples of success were about negotiating and overcoming barriers to success that had previously been too difficult to surmount. These examples were particularly important to parents, and, in many cases, as important as final outcomes of success.

Elements of success

Data analysis identified four overarching and interacting themes (or elements) about determining success, which are:

- → Final outcomes: fundamental differences or changes made for or with children and parents in parental mental health work.
- → Intermediary (process) outcomes: impacts which are associated with such changes and/or may assist in bringing final outcomes about.
- → Contributions that facilitate success: different stakeholder contributions and major opportunities to success.
- → Barriers to success, that have to be overcome or negotiated to access interventions and reach the successful outcomes described.

Figure 1: Elements of success has been developed to convey an understanding about how multiple factors within and between individuals, service providers and their environments interact. The interaction between each of the elements are illustrated by the arrows. They highlight the relevance of a systems approach to understanding the data. Each component affects, and is affected by, every other component. The key findings for each element of success are now described.

Final outcomes: safety as success (1)

The findings about 'safety as success' were not about what took place to secure 'immediate safety' of the parent or the child. Instead, they were about minimising risk and risk

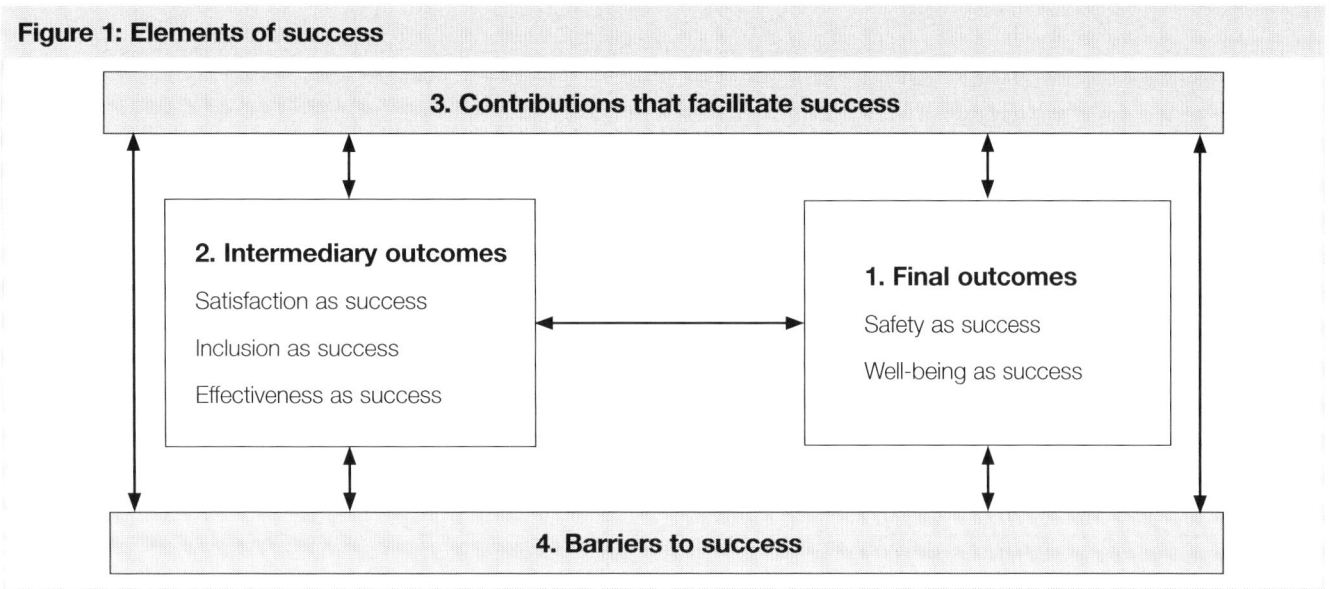

Figure 1: Elements of success

avoidance and family contributions to safety as success. These were the aspects of safeguarding that parents, children and professionals talked about.

The most prominent example of minimising and avoiding risk (highlighted by all participant groups) was the development of mental health crisis and contingency plans, and common assessment framework (CAF) and pre-CAF plans, that had been carefully constructed with parents and children and facilitated by professionals who were committed to working together and go out of their way to make it happen. Participants felt strongly that the more committed professionals were to the process and to working together, the greater the outcome achieved. Outcomes associated with the development and implementation of these plans included: a reduction in hospital admissions; shorter in-patient stays; quicker recovery times in the acute phase of illness; fewer episodes of self harm and problematic behaviour; and reduced levels of anxiety for parents and children in and out of crisis. Fully involving families in crisis and contingency planning also increased professional confidence and self-efficacy.

Assertive outreach and staying involved over time and really getting to know the family made it possible to identify safety and safeguarding concerns that had previously been missed because workers had withdrawn when initial attempts to engage the family had failed. As a consequence, families received help previously out of their reach. Outcomes tended to be short-term if intervention was short-term and family problems persisted.

Although rarer, support from extended family members to identify early signs of mental health deterioration and to mobilise support to avoid or ameliorate crisis provided a crucial element of maintaining safety and promoting well-being for parents and children. While this important source of support was recognised by professionals when it occurred, their contact with other members of the family was minimal, if any.

Interventions that have the dual focus of reducing the impact of stressors during crises and promoting the mental health and well-being of parents and children highlighted by participants included: help to understand mental illness and the impact it can have on different family members, which emerges as an extremely beneficial intervention here and in all of the elements of success; continuity in key worker; longer-term support in and out of crisis; minimal disruption of routines during a crisis; respite breaks from parenting (for parents) and from parents' difficulties (for children).

Final outcomes: well-being as success (1)

Well-being is a dynamic state that is enhanced when people can fulfil their personal and social goals. It is understood both in relation to objective measures such as household income, educational resources and health status, and subjective indicators such as happiness, perceptions of quality of life and life satisfaction. Evidence suggests that a small improvement in well-being can help to decrease some mental health problems and also help people to flourish.

Any improvement in the parent/child relationship was of high importance. Improvements occur when: parenting responsibilities are reduced; when parents have regular breaks from parenting and children have breaks from their caring responsibilities and/or exposure to their parent's difficulties. Being supported to take a holiday, listening to and playing music, dancing and being taken on a trip to the country were all ways parents and children were encouraged to appreciate how to 'stay in the moment' and appreciate 'what was happening now' as a way of freeing themselves from worries about the past and the future. Being supported financially and otherwise to engage in these pursuits was an important component in this category of success. Making new friends and having fun together was central to what works for children, as was peer support for young carers.

While parents and children experienced relationship difficulties, there was still a strong commitment by all of the parents and children to each other. Help to understand the different stages of child development and what parents need to do at each stage was also rated highly by parents. Sharing information with families in this way reduced family tension and, with support, parents and children were able to make positive adaptations in their relationships with each other, in most but not all of the case study families. This information exchange took place as part of the on-going support provided by key workers and also in the context of counselling and therapy sessions for parents, children and the whole family.

The care given by young carers, a parent's determination to keep the family together, and the willingness of family members to engage with support, were thought by everyone involved to be equally as important as service and professional contributions to success.

Young carers were proud of the role they undertook in their family and some viewed caring as a positive contributory factor to their own personal development.

Being active, feeling healthy and looking better were extremely important to all parents but this route to well-being was particularly hard to achieve and remained largely unchanged for the majority of parents taking part. Lack of energy, lack of motivation, not being able to leave the house, not being confident to attend classes on their own, not being able to afford to go swimming or to the gym were all things that parents cited as stopping them looking after themselves in this way. Children were very aware of the need to eat healthily and exercise and as a consequence worried about the impact on their parents health of not doing so.

Learning is closely entwined with well-being for adults and children and being supported to reach one academic goal emerges as a motivator to go on to achieve further success. The school environment, as a context of learning, has been found to play an important role in children's social, emotional and behavioural well-being (Gutman & Feinstein, 2008). Some children fought hard to juggle high levels of caring responsibilities with doing well academically, regardless of what was happening at home. It was clear that school provided respite and a distraction from home in these cases, but at the same time put children under continuous pressure, stepped up further, for example, during exam times or when their parent was particularly unwell. Children who were placed in schools that were a good match for a child's interests and proactively supported children in the context of their family were highly associated with a range of positive outcomes for children. Participating in service and practice development was important on a number of levels.

Parents required a lot of encouragement and support to return to education and complete courses they enrolled on. These efforts, though, were richly rewarded when a course was completed and as well as acquiring new learning and skills, their confidence and self-efficacy increased and the feelings associated with success spurred them on to do more.

Where parents and young people were encouraged to participate in service planning, research and workforce development initiatives, this resulted in a strong sense of achievement and confirmation that they had something important and worthwhile to contribute (Dolan *et al*, 2006; Hammond, 2004). There is a connection between an individual's well-being and the well-being of the wider community, and giving and sharing have a longer, more indirect association with well-being in that these types of behaviour have the potential to lead to new and stronger relationships in the future (Harlow & Cantor, 1996).

The sub-themes of safety as success and well-being as success are then intimately connected in this study about parental mental health and child welfare. They are as much about prevention, mental health promotion and promoting individual and family resilience and well-being as they are about intervening with additional support in times of crisis and taking immediate action when safety is compromised.

Intermediary outcomes: satisfaction as success (2)

This category of the findings about success relates to service user satisfaction. It casts the service user as consumer; as evaluator of the worth of the intervention. Where satisfaction is expressed in the literature, it often centres on the relationship with the worker, the worker's personal characteristics, and the provision of emotional and practical help (Cleaver *et al*, 2012; Bairstow & Hetherington, 1998; Spratt & Callan, 2004; Howe, 2008; Dale, 2004) and this is consistent with the findings in this study. Parents and children who had established a consistent trusting relationship with a professional were keen to emphasise how these relationships made a fundamental difference to the way they feel about themselves, the way they live their lives, and how these relationships were often the gateway to other successes.

Co-ordinated and inclusive care was important for those parents who experienced it, not least because their previous experience had been that services were hard to navigate and very disconnected. Help to understand mental illness was also a conduit to gaining the right kind of help. The more families and professionals understood individual and family circumstances, the more able they were to access support that worked.

Parents and children identified a number of personal and professional characteristics that they considered to be central to the successful relationships they described, and some consensus was reached about what these were. These are discussed in the section Contributions to success (see p103).

What was not apparent in the literature was the contribution that parents and children made to enable their relationships with professionals to work so well (this is also discussed under Contributions to success).

Parents and children loved to have fun and respite from their difficulties. Having fun also meant contact with other people and new situations and helped individuals and families to learn and build resilience (see also, Final outcomes: well-being as success on p99).

Intermediary outcomes: inclusion as success (2)

Success in parental mental health and child welfare work can also be detected in its application to social inclusion. Three categories of inclusion were identified in the findings: the inclusion of gaining service accessibility; the inclusion of meaningful participation; and organisational commitment to families.

The inclusion of gaining service accessibility

The findings highlight a range of intermediary actions and professional interventions that help parents and children to access services that are of best help to them. Professionals who accurately identify and match support to the needs and wishes of family members and signpost them to these made significant differences to families' lives. Statutory sector professionals did not always appreciate the significance of this important aspect of their work, though it is not clear why this was the case. One possibility might be that when a service user is signposted to another service and the case is closed by the referring agency, the referrer will not necessarily be aware of the outcome for the service user of what they have recommended. As a consequence, the success associated with the actions of these professionals, whom parents and children hold in high regard, is not known to them and opportunities to learn from their success and boost self-efficacy are diminished (Bandura, 1994).

Staying involved to support a service user through the referral process to engagement increases the take-up rate of services. Help to navigate the complex and separate systems of adult and children's services on behalf of parents and children aids access to services previously out of the family's reach.

Flexible delivery of support, for example, holding a CPA or a mental health review in a service user's home (when they are agoraphobic), or a CAF review at the school (ensuring teaching staff were present), were all ways of making sure that helpful interventions took place. A flexible approach to re-referral after a person or family have been discharged from a service helped mobilise support early, before difficulties became entrenched.

Assertive outreach was identified as a crucial element of getting support to families that may need it most. Relationships that developed through successful assertive outreach resulted in strong therapeutic bonds. Professionals argued that not working in this way results in important opportunities to intervene being missed. In some cases, safeguarding issues were identified that previous workers had missed because they had withdrawn when initial attempts to engage the family had failed (see also Final outcomes: safety as success).

Children and their parents had very different experiences of educational professionals and school environments. Children whose difficulties remained hidden for several years (which was the case for some children) and had become entrenched were more difficult to motivate and support, which is consistent with the literature (Abraham & Aldridge, 2009). Head teachers and school staff who did adopt a proactive and sensitive approach to supporting children in the context of their family supported children in a number of ways, including providing access to pastoral support at times of stress and a general willingness to treat the realities of their care-giving role as a legitimate reason on occasions when they are unable to comply with the demands placed on them at school (Eley, 2004). A very significant and additional focus for these professionals was on bridging and attending to the gap between school and home, which involved supporting parents as well as children.

The inclusion of achieving meaningful participation

This is the success of those who already have access to services and are included in information and decision-making processes regarding the services that they receive (Corby *et al*, 1996). The more parents and children participate in the assessment of their needs and care planning, the greater the incidence of success and satisfaction.

Help to provide greater understanding not only about what might be happening in the family, but also of why professionals do or say what they do, helps parents and children to understand what is being asked of them and enables them to participate more fully in decisions about their care.

Organisation commitment to families

At the time the research took place, both Liverpool and Lewisham had volunteered to be implementation sites for SCIE's *Think Child, Think Parent, Think Family* guidance (SCIE, 2009). Both have a track record of innovation in this area of practice, but Liverpool had been much more active in recent years and had a multi-agency improvement plan agreed. There was a palpable sense of pride emanating from parents, children and professionals from Liverpool who had taken part in this initiative. There were six factors, or processes, identified in the findings that appeared to support this sustained commitment to change in Liverpool. Some of these factors are consistent with the findings identified by SCIE about Liverpool as an implementation site in *Think Child, Think Parent, Think Family: Final evaluation report* (SCIE, 2012). The six factors are:

1. A group of interested and committed professionals from different agencies coming together to affect change – because services are separate and fragmented, this multi-agency approach is important if the needs of all family members are to be addressed.

2. Securing senior management involvement in the group or their 'sign up' to improvement work – senior management involvement is necessary to ensure that any improvements are firmly embedded in existing improvement agendas, to free up resources and manage implementation and evaluation in collaboration with other managers – identifying and securing the membership of all necessary parties is crucial to this success factor.

3. A commitment to evidence-based decision making (drawing on the best available evidence from research, practice, and service user and carer expertise) – researching local need, ensuring new developments are independently evaluated and volunteering to be implementation sites for SCIE's *Think Child, Think Parent, Think Family* guidance (SCIE, 2009) were all ways of contributing not only to the local evidence base about what works, but also the national policy and practice agenda (SCIE, 2012).

4. A strong commitment to co-production and participation from the outset ensuring that families are involved and supported in all aspects of service development and review – this was firmly developed in Liverpool and part of mainstream service development practice and was facilitated by Barnardo's Action with Young Carers project. It was less developed in Lewisham at the time of the research.

5. Being willing to tackle the 'too difficult to handle' issues that had previously been set aside – choosing to tackle some of the 'too difficult to handle issues' that had the most potential to effect families and challenge staff increased local confidence in the ability of senior management group to achieve positive change.

6. Recording and sharing 'what works' locally and nationally – by communicating their successes via publications and at local and national events; contributing their expertise to new policy developments; delivering training and consultancy across the country; and formal evaluation of their work. Thus contributing further to the evidence base about 'what works'.

This 'top down, bottom up' approach to change has resulted in significant and sustained changes in Liverpool. The senior management group involved in this work, which has grown in numbers over time, includes representation from: the local authority (CSC, Young Carers, Education); the mental health trust (adult and child and adolescence); public health; health and social care commissioning groups; a number of voluntary sector agencies and service user representatives. The membership are clear that the cornerstone of their success is the combined sum and nature of the people involved, and that the work undertaken would be seen by others as 'over and above' what their organisation requires of their substantive posts. Therefore, if members of the group leave, the sustainability of the group and the work becomes threatened. In recognition of this, the group aim to mainstream the processes and resources that they develop to increase their survival rate – by embedding changes into everyday practice. In contrast to Liverpool, Lewisham struggled to secure sufficient senior management commitment to the improvement work that they been planned and as a consequence change was patchy and slow.

Intermediary outcomes: effectiveness as success (2)

Effectiveness as success is about interventions and service models positively evaluated by parents, children and professionals as examples of what had worked for them.

Social care interventions that have the potential to break the cycle of deprivation that all of the families in this study experienced were the hardest for families to access and achieve, for example, unemployment, poor housing and poverty. These were the circumstances that parents, children and professionals felt had the most power to change families' lives but were the most difficult to attain and sustain. There were, however, examples of services that aimed to intervene early to break down the cycle of impacts that can occur across the lifespan and generation that had been very successful, such as helping young people increase their chances for employment and facilitating school transitions.

Being able to benefit from any intervention was influenced by who was recommending or delivering the intervention, what else was happening for the family at the time of the intervention, what other interventions were happening concurrently, and the timeliness, timing and duration of the intervention.

Interventions that contribute to success

Interventions to improve mental health, particularly psychiatric medication, were thought by children and professionals to be very important and were associated with a number of positive outcomes for parents, children and the whole family (see Contributions to success). However, tensions arise from this, as while the majority of parents could see that taking medication helped, it did not provide anything like the relief they hoped for. The requirement for most of the parents to keep taking medication as a prophylactic to prevent breakthrough symptoms, and the adverse affects associated with some medications, were sometimes too difficult to bear – particularly when they believed that the need for treatment might be significantly reduced or stopped if improvements could be made in other areas of their lives (e.g. poor housing, poverty, isolation). So, while the aim to promote mental health in this way is entirely laudable and commendable, it is not without its costs to parents.

Where professionals and parents were committed to working together to review the effectiveness of medication and optimise its effects, sometimes for lengthy periods of time, the rewards included maximisation of treatment outcomes, reduced side effects, improved compliance and better mental health for longer periods – which was beneficial for parents and children. Community psychiatric nurses (CPNs) adopted a bio-psychosocial approach to explaining: how medication works; why a 'therapeutic level' has to be reached; why stopping medication abruptly can be detrimental; why drinking alcohol or taking illegal substances can reduce the effect of medication and exacerbate side effects or symptoms; and why some medications help some people in some situations and not others. This was very highly valued by parents who had engaged with their CPN to do this work.

A range of interventions targeted to promote resilience and reduce stressors identified in the findings are consistent with research evidence. For example, young carers interventions, including peer support, focusing on the whole family, respite from caring opportunities and the availability of a trusted adult to talk to and help with school transitions (Dearden & Becker, 2004; Grant *et al*, 2008). Taking part in a young carer's assessment and being acknowledged as a young carer emerged as an important way of helping to validate and contextualise young people's experiences (Roberts & Wolfson, 2006).

Regular respite opportunities and supported holidays and breaks for young people and whole families that were financed by the voluntary sector and sometimes CMHTs enabled parents and children to have a break from their surroundings and circumstances and experience different things. The value of looked after/respite care has been corroborated by research (Aldgate & Bradley, 1999; Packman & Hall, 1998; Greenfields & Statham, 2004) (see Safety as success).

Spending time with other parents or young people with similar experiences, hearing their stories and what they found worked for them, helped parents and children to feel less isolated and more able to try new strategies for change.

Regular encouragement from key workers who consistently conveyed their belief in what parents and children could achieve was central to helping parents and children overcome self-doubt, take risks, and begin to identify what they need to do and what else needs to happen to not only cope with their circumstances but to recover and live well. There were also examples of this reinforcement and encouragement occurring in counselling and family therapy.

Service models that contribute to success

The findings in this study are consistent with the idea that families affected by parental mental illness and multiple disadvantages may need a multi-dimensional approach and range of interventions over a longer period of time (Dearden & Becker, 2004; Grant *et al*, 2008; Aked *et al*, 2008; Foresight, 2008; Bartley, 2006). Neighbourhood services, where parents and children form a relationship with the centre as a whole and where an 'episodic' service is available which is consistent with approach offered by the voluntary sector agencies taking part in this research appear as particularly appropriate for families with long-term problems, including recurring mental illness which is consistent with the literature (Thoburn *et al*, 2000).

Contributions to success (3)

Parents, children and professionals were asked to identify their contribution to the successful situations they had described. They were also asked to describe other people's contributions to success and any opportunities that had arisen that helped to facilitate the positive outcomes they described.

Parents, children and other family member contributions

Without exception, children identified as the most important contribution that parents could make to success was 'taking their medication' (see also Intermediary outcomes: effectiveness as success on p102).

Parents described their most important contribution to success as 'keeping their family together,' despite the difficulties experienced by themselves and their families.

A parent's ability to overcome the stigma associated with statutory services and the suspicion and mistrust borne of previous failures to get support for themselves and their families was also identified as an important component of success Asking for help required a great deal of emotional energy and commitment which some parents and children felt they did not have to give. The lasting and painful impact of previous and repeated rejections when they had sought help, coupled with the stigma associated with seeking help from CSC and mental health services, left parents and children wary of committing themselves to a relationship with a new professional.

Parents and children were extremely willing to give and give back to their peers and the agencies that they were working with and there were many examples of the significant contributions they had made.

Children are extremely loyal to their parents and fiercely protective of them. This, and the positive attitude that most young carers adopted, helped children to understand their situation more readily, and, as a number of children said, 'just get on with it'. However, this stoicism can mask significant unmet need.

Emotional and practical support provided by extended family members, friends and the church provided a crucial contribution to promoting safety and well-being for the few families who benefitted from this.

Parents and children are clear and unanimous about the personal and professional characteristics that they associate with best professional practice, and professionals agree. Parents, children and other professionals (of each other) say they value professionals who:

- are genuinely interested in them and care about them, not just about their problems
- are flexible and willing to work outside of what would be considered normative professional boundaries (e.g. hold a review meeting at home; phoning them at the weekend)
- offer them enough time to talk, get to know them well and can then see things from their perspective
- are reliable, do what they say they are going to and are available when they are needed
- don't give up or forget them even when parents/children/families turn them away
- are knowledgeable and skilled in ways that can help them with their difficulties and can provide opportunities otherwise out of their reach
- are fair, honest and are prepared to challenge them (this was commented only by parents and children who thought professionals had taken the time to get to know them well) as well as offer support in a non-judgmental way
- stay with them in and out of crisis and overtime
- are willing to tackle and work with other agencies and bureaucratic systems (such as service eligibility thresholds) on their behalf
- (for parents) continue to think about and support their children when they cannot
- help them to reflect on and address their difficulties by sharing information they have gained from their professional training and practice experience
- persevere, don't give up and are willing to go the extra mile.

These characteristics were present in different combinations in the professionals that parents, children and other professionals cited as making a very significant contribution to success.

Professionals described a number of sources that they drew upon to support their practice: their own family experiences of mental health helped them understand what families were experiencing; professional training and high-quality professional supervision (Katz et al, 2007); and importantly being curious, learning from experience, from service users, and from professionals from other disciplines. CMHT professionals valued the expertise that was available to them via their multi-disciplinary team and the ethos and culture of the voluntary sector organisations allowed them to do things that were not similarly supported in the statutory agencies (e.g. assertive outreach and the length of time they were able to spend with clients). Professional practice was best supported when organisations allowed and encouraged professionals to go at the pace of the family, and to be flexible and stay involved for the long-term if needed.

Barriers to success (4)

Unsurprisingly, many examples in the findings about final and intermediary outcomes of success were about overcoming the obstacles described in the research data and the literature about barriers to success.

Helping the child versus supporting the parent is a dilemma that affects all agencies. Despite high levels of agency involvement over time with each of the families interviewed, the focus for intervention and support gravitated to the parent. All of the children believed that their parent needed lots of help, but older children on the whole felt aggrieved that there was not more help available for themselves, while younger children felt that because their parent was ill and it was not their fault, it was right that they should have the most help.

Children hid the extent of their own difficulties from their parents and professionals because they did not want their parents to feel more guilty or for services to intervene and separate them from their parents.

Some (but not all) parents had minimised the issues that gave concern to child social care (CSC) and other agencies over time, for example concerns about neglect, emotional abuse and parental substance misuse. There was evidence on statutory agency case files of an overreliance by professionals on what parents have to say about their children's difficulties. It was also clear that other significant adult/parent carers and children in the family were not routinely consulted by any of the agencies concerned, with the exception of crisis situations. The significance of these omissions becomes more apparent when looking at the data from the individual interviews, where children clearly described the impact of their parent's difficulties on themselves as far greater than what their parents described in their interviews or than what they disclosed to professionals, as described in the case file records.

Little attention was paid to other children in the family unless they had presented with difficulties of their own that were being supported by services.

Extended family members were not routinely contacted, supported or involved in assessment and care planning processes by any of the agencies involved; neither were they included in any safeguarding or well-being goals.

Professionals were not always aware of, or took steps to find out, who else was working with the family, and all of the agency case files had gaps in information about the assessment and activities of other agencies.

Difficulties gathering and analysing the breadth and depth of information needed to get a comprehensive picture of the family's history and current functioning were apparent on case files. A gap was identified in how the details of past history – particularly as determinants of future risk and current knowledge – are recorded and utilised in assessments and care planning. There was evidence to suggest that this information was not always understood or used to asses risk or identify opportunities for prevention for young children in the family.

Managers and practitioners (from all professional groups) who lack confidence and have insufficient knowledge about adult and child mental health and child development may avoid asking 'difficult questions' or talking to children because they are wary of stigmatising parents or making things worse.

CSC are increasingly perceived as focusing on assessing current safety and paying insufficient attention to future safety, largely because of increasing demand on their service. This was particularly the case in assessment and responses to children's emotional needs, which did not include enough attention to the impact over time of continuous or frequent intermittent exposure to parental difficulties on children's mental health and well-being. Lack of CSC oversight or periodic reassessment also leads to the 'start again' again approach that many families experience.

There were unacceptably long waiting periods for referrals between agencies that resulted in a decrease in service users' motivation to take part, and in several cases the resource did not materialise at all. This is included waiting for resources deemed as essential in Children's Safeguarding plans.

Professionals (schools in particular) not taking parents' and children's concerns seriously and not having sufficient knowledge about child mental health issues (all professional groups) meant that children with significant emotional, mental health or behavioural problems and caring responsibilities remain unidentified for very long periods.

Conclusion

Conceptualising success

There are a number of interrelated factors that can make it difficult to conceptualise, identify, work towards and evaluate, success. These include: a preoccupation with avoiding failure rather than focusing on success; being conditioned to learn from mistakes and not success; practitioners doubting their contribution to success; and a preoccupation that more could be done but resources do not permit this, and so there is nothing to be done. On the other hand, there are agencies, managers and professionals who are curious and willing to learn from the experience of families, other professionals and from their day-to-day experience of working with individuals and families. They are the ones who negotiate and overcome the barriers to success.

This study has put the concept of success at the core of working with parental mental health and child welfare. It has demonstrated that success not only happens, but is recognised by parents and children as a source for further positive change. It enables a move from a one-dimensional perspective of parents as deficits carriers, to include dimensions such as their strengths, their ability to be change agents for themselves and their children, and to recognise the need for a more holistic conceptual framework to this area including paying attention to other aspects of parents lives. This links well with the conceptual frameworks of the new meaning of recovery and particularly of mental health promotion (Ralph & Corrigan 2005; Friedli, 2009).

The research has identified parents and children's contributions to 'what works', which is largely missing from the existing literature (with the exception of young carers). It has also identified the important contribution that effective user participation makes to service user outcomes, the outcomes of other service users, and to practice development and research.

Methodological contribution

The exploratory nature of this study has enabled a rich and contextualised picture of the different elements of success and pathways to success to emerge. The incorporation of different stakeholder groups has allowed the findings to be grounded in the experiences of parents, children and professionals.

The choice of data collection methods, and the presentation of allowing the findings from the first phase of data collection to be used for discussion by key stakeholders in the second phase, has enabled fresh insights to be gained about this topic, including new contributions to our understanding of the dilemmas that families and professionals experience in this service context and their responses to these dilemmas.

Focusing on multiple perspectives, enables the applicability of the findings to be relevant to all of the participant groups taking part.

Potential contributions to practice

A primary objective of the research was to explore whether the key participants in parental mental health and child welfare work share methods and practices that could be distilled and disseminated for wider exploration and application. It has, in fact, turned out that while the practitioners' work associated with success in this study differed from the work of many of their colleagues, there are similarities in their attitudes and approaches to the families whom they helped. The research explicates, on the basis of these similarities, a mode of working that seems to make it possible to succeed in helping many families previously considered beyond help or whom others have struggled to help.

Training to work with success at the core of practice

This is an exploratory study, hence the organisation and practice principles identified are distilled as a first step in developing a body of practice knowledge for others who will be working with families where there is a parent with mental illness.

The limitations of the study

Several limitations have been identified. The sample is too small to enable generalisation. It is also skewed by having more participants from Liverpool, despite the efforts to widen the sample pool. All but two of the children/young people taking part were young carers, who are not representative of other sub-groups of children in families. However, for an exploratory study such as this one, it is more important to understand and portray the views of the different groups of participants (Ramon *et al*, 2007) than to attempt generalisation based on less in-depth study.

Not all case study family members were recruited to take part in the research, and the professionals involved were limited to the agencies recruited to the study, some of which were already seen as 'exemplars' in this area of practice and therefore not necessarily typical of similar agencies in other areas. Some children in families were not invited to take part because they were too young, were not living at home, or experienced difficulties that being interviewed might exacerbate. In some families more than one child was receiving services, and in two of the families I was able to interview two children from each. There were no fathers referred to in the study, largely because there were far fewer fathers engaged with the agencies taking part in the research and there were none that met the criteria for inclusion.

There were a number of other family members in the case study families whose perspectives might have enhanced the case studies further, including:

- → fathers who were still supporting and caring for their children but living separately
- → adult partners living at home and sharing the care of the children
- → other children in the family that had not been referred to services
- → grandparents who helped to look after their grandchildren and were closely supporting their child (the parent)
- → teachers and learning mentors whose involvement was particularly significant for some children
- → CAMHS staff who had supported a number of young people who had experienced emotional and behavioural difficulties.

However, this information has become known only after the study has taken place and is dependent on the circumstances of each family, rather than there being a particular missing group that is relevant to all families. It was possible in response to the above to include CAMHS representation on the professional focus group.

Future research

The findings of this exploratory study could be used as the basis for a longitudinal study that would follow the pathway to success of a greater number, and more representative sample, of families in order to gather sufficient data with a large enough representative sample to demonstrate the effectiveness of researching success for this specific population. This would strengthen the evidence base, and may impact on professionals and policy makers to consider success as a core element in the work with this group.

Emotional and practical support provided by extended family members and friends, where it is available, can provide a crucial contribution to promoting safety and well-being. However, professionals from all sectors appear reluctant to engage other members of the family or include them in safeguarding and well-being goals. Further research is suggested to explore these different perspectives in order to gain further insights about success and about how these perspectives can be harnessed by professionals.

Education, schools, school processes and staff actions featured highly in the findings about success and barriers to success. There were some very strong examples in the research about how, when schools intervene and support children and their parents successfully, this can lead to positive and far-reaching outcomes. Learning more about these successes, what helps to facilitate them and their applicability to other school settings, could be an important contribution to knowledge and practice in schools and ultimately lead to earlier identification and support for children.

Final thoughts

This is the first study to focus on multiple perspectives of success with this specific population. By putting the concept of success at the core of working with parental mental health and child welfare, it has demonstrated that success not only happens, but is recognised by parents and children as a source of further positive change.

Many of the practice principles identified are not new and will be seen by many practitioners as a statement of what good social care and health practice has always been about. Or they can be seen as a preliminary map of a territory which can be further explored and refined, which is most compatible to the research philosophy underpinning this research.

An examination of emerging themes and the interplay between themes gives insight into the shared ideas about what works and the shared methods and practices that are associated with successful outcomes. On the basis of these similarities, the findings offer a contribution to knowledge and practice about a mode of working that seems to make it possible to succeed in helping families previously considered difficult to help. What is more, the practitioners also benefit from the helping relationship in this context.

References

Abraham K & Aldridge J (2009) *The Mental Wellbeing of Young Carers in Manchester.* Manchester Carers Forum: Manchester.

Aked J, Marks N, Thompson S & Cordon C (2008) *Five Ways to Wellbeing.* London: New Economics Foundation.

Aldgate J & Bradley M (1999) *Supporting Families Through Short Term Fostering.* London: The Stationery Office.

Bairstow K & Hetherington R (1998) Parents' experiences of child welfare interventions: an Anglo-French comparison. *Child and Society* **12** pp113–114.

Bandura A (1994) Self-efficacy. In: VS Ramachaudran (2012) *Encyclopedia of Human Behaviour* (pp71–81). New York: Academic Press.

Bartley M (2006) *Capability and Resilience: Beating the odds* [online]. London: ESRC Human Capability and Resilience Research Network. Available at: www.ucl.ac.uk/capabilityandresilience (accessed November 2015).

Brandon M & Thoburn J (2008) Safeguarding children in the UK: a longitudinal study of services to children suffering or likely to suffer significant harm. *Child and Family Social Work* **13** pp365–377.

Cleaver H, Unell I & Aldgate J (2012) *Children's Needs: Parenting capacity* (2nd edition). London: DfE TSO.

Corby B, Millar M & Young L (1996) Parental participation in child protection work: rethinking the rhetoric. *British journal of social work* **26** pp475–492.

Dale P (2004) Like a fishbowl: parents' perceptions of child protection interventions. *Child Abuse Review* **13** pp137–157.

Dearden C & Becker S (2004) *Young Carers in the UK: the 2004 report.* London: Carers UK and The Children's Society.

Dolan P, Peasgood T & White M (2006) *Review of Research on the Influences on Personal Wellbeing and Application to Policy Making.* London: Defra.

Eley S (2004) 'If they don't recognise it, you've got to deal with it yourself': gender, young caring and education support. *Gender & education* **16** (1) pp65–75.

Foresight (2008) *Foresight Mental Capital and Wellbeing Project.* London: The Government Office for Science.

Friedli L (2009) *Mental Health, Resilience and Inequalities.* London: World Health Organisation, Mental Health Foundation.

Grant G, Repper J & Nolan M (2008) Young people supporting parents with mental health problems: experiences of assessment and support. *Health and Social Care in the Community* **16** pp271–281.

Greenfields H & Statham J (2004) *Support Foster Care: Developing a short break service for children in need.* London: Thomas Coram Research Unit.

Gutman LM & Feinstein L (2008) *Children's Wellbeing in Primary School: Pupil and school effects.* London: Centre for Research on the Wider Benefits of Learning: Institute of Education.

Hammond C (2004) Impacts of lifelong learning upon emotional resilience, psychological and mental health: fieldwork evidence. *Oxford review of education* **30** 551–568.

Harlow RE & Cantor N (1996) Still participating after all these years: a study of life task participation in later life. *Journal of Personality and Social Psychology* **71** 1235–1249.

Howe D (2004) *The Emotionally Intelligent Social Worker.* Basingstoke: Palgrave Macmillan.

Katz I (2007) Community interventions for vulnerable children and families. *Communities Children & Families* **3** (1) pp19–32.

Katz I & Pinkerton J (Eds) (2003) *Seeking Effective Interventions for Young Offenders: Interim results of a four-year randomized study of multisystemic therapy in Onrtario Canada.* London, Ontario: Centre for Children and Families in the Justice System.

Kim-Cohen J (2003) Prior juvenile diagnoses in adults with mental disorder: developmental follow-back of a prospective longitudinal cohort. *Archives of general psychiatry* **60** pp709–717.

Packman J & Hall C (1998) *From Care to Accommodation.* London: The Stationary Office.

Ralph R & Corrigan P (2005) *Recovery in Mental Illness: Broadening our understanding of wellness.* Washington: American Psychological Association.

Ramon S, Healy B & Renouf N (2007) Recovery from mental illness as an emergent concept and practice in Australia and the UK. *International Journal of Social Psychiatry* **53** (2) p108–122.

Roberts G & Wolfson P (2006) *The Rediscovery of Recovery: Open to all – advances in psychiatric treatment.* London: The Royal College of Psychiatrists.

Rutter M & Quinton D (1984) Parental psychiatric disorder: effects on children. *Psychological medicine* **14** pp853–880.

SCIE (2009) *Think Child, Think Parent, Think Family: A guide to parental mental health and child welfare.* London: Social Care Institute for Excellence.

SCIE (2012) *Report 56: Think Child, Think Parent, Think Family: Final evaluation report.* London: Social Care Institute for Excellence.

Spratt T & Callan J (2004) Parents' views on social work interventions in child welfare cases. *British Journal of Social Work* **34** (2) pp199–224.

Thoburn J, Chand A & Proctor J (2000) *Child Welfare Services for Minority Ethnic Families: The research reviewed.* London: Jessica Kingsley.

Yin RK (2003) *Case Study Research: Design and methods.* London: Sage.

# Chapter 16

Success in safeguarding children in the UK

By Andy Quin

Introduction

In this chapter I draw on the findings from an exploratory case study of success and collaboration in safeguarding work that was conducted between 2010 and 2013 in one local area in the UK. This qualitative study started from the assumption that participants in safeguarding practice hold knowledge about success, including children, parents and practitioners, as well as connected others such as family members, those who supervise and manage practitioners and those who commission and regulate services. Because these participants play very different roles in the operation of a safeguarding system and have different interests, we cannot assume that they are driven by the same idea of success. Gaining an understanding of success in safeguarding therefore requires getting close to practice and studying what participants say and do.

Why focusing on success is important

Success is rarely studied in safeguarding work. We are all more familiar with reports of atrocities towards children and negligence on the part of professionals or services than we are of stories of success. Where there are calls for learning from experience, these are mainly about learning from mistakes. Although current government guidance recognises the importance of identifying and sharing good practice (HM Government, 2015), the content of its advice is almost entirely about learning from error, principally through mechanisms such as serious case reviews. There is also a tendency for those involved in researching safeguarding work to focus more on problematic practice rather than examples of success. For example, in searching through databases of the many reports and journal articles on safeguarding children, it is difficult to find studies that focus specifically on successes. This is not to say that studying mistakes is unimportant, indeed it is vital to look carefully and respectfully for lessons when children are fatally or seriously harmed and safeguarding services have been involved. However, there are three main arguments as to why the search for mistakes should be balanced by a quest for success.

The first of these concerns understanding what success means in safeguarding work. We have become used to seeing success as safety or the absence of significant harm to the child involved. While the absence of maltreatment is a vital foundation to be sought in safeguarding work, it is a limited and insufficient aim by itself. Complementary goals are needed that relate to the potential for intervention to facilitate growth, development and well-being. There may be agreement on what constitutes an absence of maltreatment to a child, but beyond this criterion of success, different opinions exist on what well-being, for example, means. Attending to diverse perspectives on success strengthens our ability to evaluate safeguarding activity.

The second argument is about human rights and respect for the person. Safeguarding is often exercised in the name of the human rights of the child, but it must be practised in ways that respect the human rights of all involved. Respect for human rights includes consideration for individual capacities: for the practitioner's, parent's or child's capacity to deliberate, to make choices, to act and to realise their goals. Clearly, there are boundaries in focusing on human agency in this way, and some choices and actions may be injurious to the capacities and freedoms of others. Nevertheless, attention to achievements and successes is an essential part of humane safeguarding practice.

The third argument relates to the learning potential arising from studying success. Based on their study of collective learning in schools, Schechter *et al* (2008) note the inherent threat involved in acknowledging mistakes, where practitioners can engage in denial and avoidance concerning evaluations of their actions. By contrast, learning from successful events is associated with increases in confidence, motivation, and in shared beliefs about the capacity to succeed in the future. These potential gains are not restricted to particular institutions such as schools, nor confined just to the work of individuals or groups of professionals; the potential of learning from success applies to both safeguarding practitioners and family members alike.

In one sense, searching for success is a straightforward exercise. The pages of government guidance provide what may be called the normative view of success in safeguarding children, emphasising the safety of children as indicated by decisions on child protection plans. Success from this perspective can be measured and tracked by changes in numbers or rates per 10,000 children; by the duration of plans or by the numbers of children who experience second or additional periods of being subject to these plans. This normative view is also contained in the reports of those who regulate and inspect safeguarding services. Success here is reflected in the attainment of standards considered by regulators to be necessary for the safety and well-being of children. In another sense, these conceptions of success are narrow and anchored to organisational processes rather than outcomes for people (Tilbury, 2004). However, this normative view provides no understanding of success as a lived experience of those directly involved in safeguarding work.

A study of success

The following findings come from PhD research in the form of a multiple embedded case study in one local area of England (Bluechester). The case study aimed to understand the perspectives of different participants in safeguarding work and it focused on three practice settings. The first of these concerned accounts of safeguarding work with individual children who had been subject to a child protection plan. A small number of parents and social workers were interviewed about their experiences of safeguarding interventions. Written accounts of interventions were also read from case records. The second setting involved the work of two safeguarding teams in Bluechester and the third setting concerned the activity of Bluechester's local safeguarding children board (LSCB). In both settings, data was collected through ethnographic observation in team workplaces and LSCB meetings as well as through a review of documents. All sets of data were thematically analysed.

Success in safeguarding takes multiple and dynamic forms

In Bluechester, multiple forms of success coexisted within the same local system for safeguarding children (Figure 1). From the practitioners' perspective, success was found in coping with crises, in winning the confidence of parents and young people, and in reaching performance targets. Parents found success in feeling vindicated following accusations of abuse or in obtaining sought after services for their children. Success was found in emotional and relational improvements in the lives of children and parents. Managers, meanwhile, found success in performance improvements and in meeting the expectations of the regulator.

Safeguarding intervention gives rise to large and small successes. Micro-successes are identified by practitioners or parents. Safeguarding also prompts broader, more reflective evaluations of past interventions and their impact over time. Achievements are recognised with respect to either general or highly specific aspects of children's lives: to the individual child's safety or the safety of a cohort of children; to holistic improvement for a child, or to improvements in particular aspects of well-being such as diet, weight or social relationships. These differences of focus stem in part from the different roles and interests at play in safeguarding work – for example between managers, practitioners and family members.

Bluechester parents who were interviewed valued their autonomy, respect from others and also the availability of practical support from local services. Practitioners, on the other hand, looked for engagement by children and parents, a working understanding of the family's life and the child's experience within it. Both practitioners and managers placed value on the completion of tasks and actions. Beyond this, managers had the challenging task of rationalising service demand within available resources, of limiting costs and improving quality. There were potential victories in each of these areas but also potential conflicts of interest.

Improvements in the child's welfare and safety represented an achievement for all parties in Bluechester. However, beyond this there were other objects of success. The reputation and good standing of safeguarding services represented a further field for success. Criticism by inspectors and regulators represented a powerful threat for local organisations with safeguarding responsibilities. Much activity within the LSCB was therefore expended on scrutinising progress against critical inspection reports, auditing and monitoring data on the extent

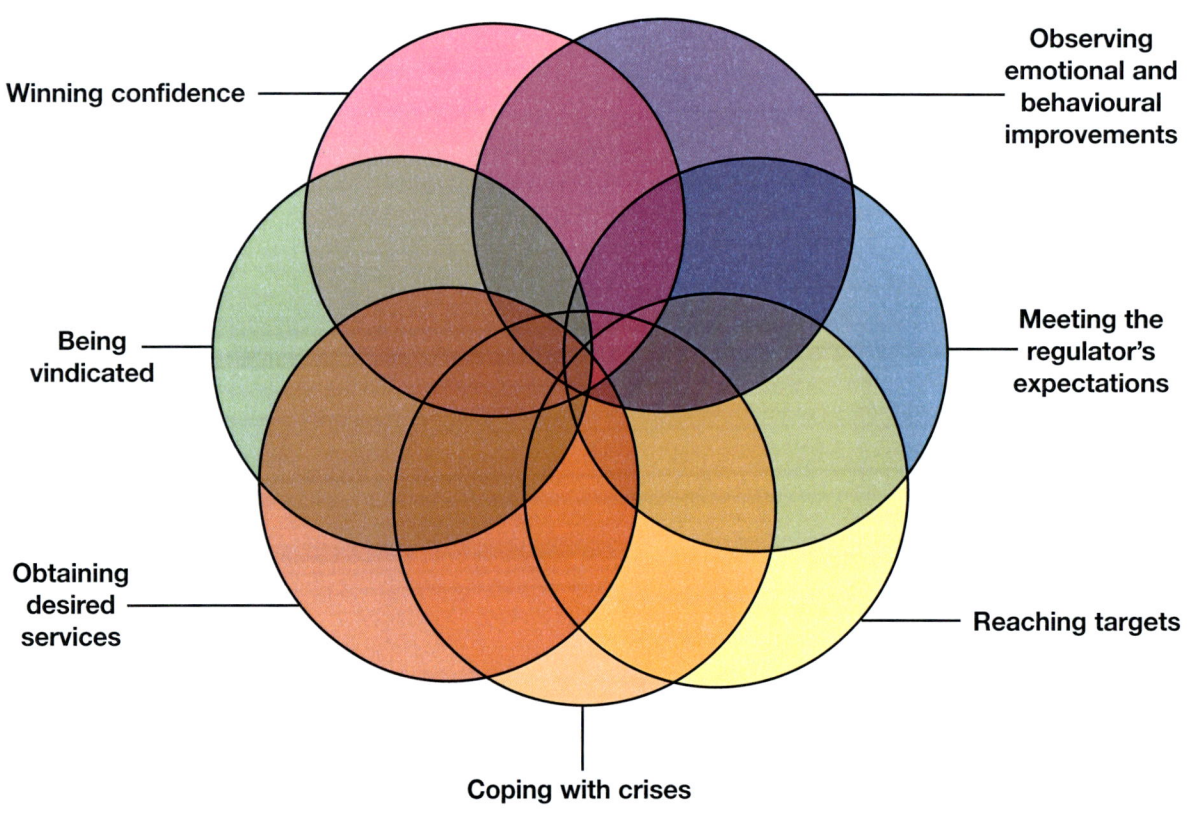

Figure 1: Multiple and intersecting success

of compliance with service standards valued by regulators. For managers of services, improved standards represented success. This was not only associated with improved outcomes for children but also with organisational survival.

Safeguarding participants therefore have varied interests and differences of focus. There is the child to think about, but also the organisation and the self. The coexistence of these different objects and forms of success provides a multi-layered experience. Safeguarding intervention can generate satisfaction from relational improvements and, at the same time, evoke the pleasure of having redressed an injustice. Coexisting evaluations may be congruent and inter-relate positively, or may conflict and produce dissonance. For example, intervention may be perceived to bring about positive change in a child's life during a period when regulators have branded local safeguarding services as inadequate.

Success is not only a multi-layered experience but also a dynamic one. Evaluations of safeguarding are subject to rapid change. Success can come and go with new events in children's and parents' lives: the success of withstanding a crisis is dissolved with the onset of a new one; additional information may cause reinterpretations and question previous evaluations of progress. Success, as a transitory experience, is fostered also by the constant change of practitioners allocated to cases due to staff shortages and by the drive for continual improvement. Stories of success can become buried in case records or be lost as one practitioner working with a family is replaced by another. The achievement of meeting targets is short-lived as new goals and challenges are constantly set.

A dominating 'success'

In Bluechester, the dominant form of success was one that might be termed 'avoiding failure'. The failure to be avoided is harm or maltreatment to the child, and particularly harm that may be attributable in some measure to errors, misjudgement or negligence by safeguarding services and practitioners. Harm to the child in this sense also means harm to the organisation and the self. The search for this success was marked by a priority on surveillance of risk to children, risk screening by managers and legal advisors, and earlier steps to formalise intervention and use care proceedings. It was also seen in the emphasis on audits and the concern for compliance with targets and procedures.

This form of success was dominant in Bluechester in the sense that the priority given to targets and standards trumped other forms of success. Practitioners could be observed making arrangements to visit families out of a concern for meeting performance timescales. Similarly, what seemed like reasonable requests by parents to reschedule child protection conferences to enable them to be present were refused due to concerns about the impact on performance metrics. In such examples, the powerful drive to avoid organisational failure appears to work against attaining a success associated with participation and meaningful engagement with families. In these ways, this concern to avoid failure and the actions associated with its promotion represent a form of defensive practice (Harris, 1987). Harris argues that defensive practices, such as the generation of extensive procedures, arise out of an institutional fear of child abuse tragedies, but have consequences that actually work against the well-being of children for whom there are concerns. However, in the current context it is not just the fear of the child abuse tragedy but also the fear of the regulator that fosters this defensiveness.

Avoiding failure in safeguarding work involves selective attention to gaps, deficiencies and problems – in the lives of children and parents, in the activities of practitioners, and in the operation of organisations. While problem-solving is a necessary part of safeguarding work, a remorseless hunt for failures and inadequacies results in a blindness to what is going well. Avoiding failure is also associated with a confidence in the top-down application of improvement measures. These strategies are likely to have limited impact as they largely ignore the contribution of those most involved: practitioners and family members who themselves have knowledge and wisdom about positive change. The belief that all participants in safeguarding have strengths, and the reorientation to pay attention to successes as well failures, provides more solid basis for improvement. As Berg and Kelly put it:

> *'Any time, place, or situation that the person could have done drugs, drank, slapped, cursed, or left a child unsupervised, but somehow managed not to, is a treasure chest of resources to build on. Instead of brushing off such small, seemingly insignificant successes, pay attention to the details of how the caretaker managed to avoid lashing out at the child. These can become the building blocks of bigger successes in the future.'* (Berg & Kelly, 2000, p104)

Shared success

Featherstone *et al* (2014) have cautioned about a child-centred approach to safeguarding work, which effectively de-couples the child from their family; one that treats the child as a separate legal entity with an independent relation to the state. The concern is that this orientation atomises the child. It diminishes their complex relational self and their social identities. Effectively, it excludes the possibility of a success in safeguarding work that the child and other family members share together.

This was very recognisable in Bluechester. The records and interviews of social workers showed that their gaze was firmly on the child within the family. Where a relationship with parents had been established, this orientation was accompanied by an understanding of the parent's world. Where no relationship had been established or it had broken down, parents had only an instrumental importance. Only their actions counted. Their subjectivity, their hopes and achievements, were unknown and unrecorded. On the one hand, interviewed parents were able to identify safeguarding achievements arising from their own actions and how these benefited their child and themselves. On the other hand, practitioners and their organisations worked within a framework for recording outcomes that focused on the child alone. Similarly, at a strategic level, the Bluechester LSCB monitored only child-related data – performance indicators concerning, for example, children referred to social care services, assessments undertaken on children, and children with child protection plans. The LSCB had no formal mechanisms to consult children and family members and thus no means of exploring the views and narratives of children and parents who had experienced safeguarding interventions.

Learning from success in safeguarding children

Given that there are significant differences in the way success is experienced, learning from it requires some choices and definitions about what and whose success we are learning from. There is a pathway for learning the success encouraged by regulators and statutory guidance. This includes inter-organisational learning where management knowledge is transferred from those with outstanding inspection reports and excellent performance metrics to organisations requiring improvement. This learning is about strengthening the managerial grip on practice – ways of ensuring, for example, that a greater proportion of child protection plans are complete within an 18 to 24 month window and cases are systematically screened by managers and lawyers for the early application of care proceedings. The government has actively encouraged this sort of learning. It is exampled by peer review arrangements between local authorities in which the quality and performance of children's services are examined and recommendations made.

Alternatively, we can learn from parents who manage to keep their children safe and promote their welfare despite multiple adversities such as poor health, low income or housing deprivation, or parents who manage against the odds to obtain support from hard-to-reach services: services that are difficult to access or that respond to budget reductions by raising thresholds for provision. This learning is partly about resilience, and partly about how parents, as active agents, utilise their strengths to safeguard their children. There is much to learn in this field and current knowledge of this form of success appears fragmented. There are some studies of parents' or families' successes (Lietz, 2006; 2007; 2009; Richter & Bammer, 2000) and more personal narrative accounts of survivors found in blogs or website forums.

Finally, we can learn from the success of practitioners, parents, young people and family members who, in the context of concerns about maltreatment, have worked together to produce beneficial change. There is already a body of knowledge to draw on. This emphasises the importance of the relationship in child welfare work generally, including practice where maltreatment is an issue. This knowledge includes findings from studies of what children and parents find helpful in relationships with practitioners (Dale, 2004; Morgan, 2006; Buckley et al, 2010; Ribner & Knei-Paz, 2002), and knowledge of methodologies of work in safeguarding situations, including practices emphasising the strengths rather than deficiencies of family members (Berg & Kelly, 2000; Saleebey, 2009; Turnell & Edwards, 1997; Kemp et al, 2014).

Each of these pathways for learning (summarised in Figure 2) is important in developing an understanding of what success means in safeguarding children. Quality services are important. It is right that effort is expended on developing and maintaining standards of practice, although in achieving this there is a balance to be struck between management control and the forms of self-regulation associated with highly skilled, knowledgeable and committed practitioners with a strong professional identity.

And quality services are only one side of the equation. We also need to acknowledge and build a better understanding of the role parents and family members play in safeguarding children and how this agency can be supported by services that are accessible, available in quantity as well as quality, and respectful in terms of the needs of those requiring them. Finally, there is more to learn from the interaction of these contributions. Particularly in situations where the agency of parents is under-developed or exhausted, skilled relational help can promote the confidence, motivation and the exercise of their strengths.

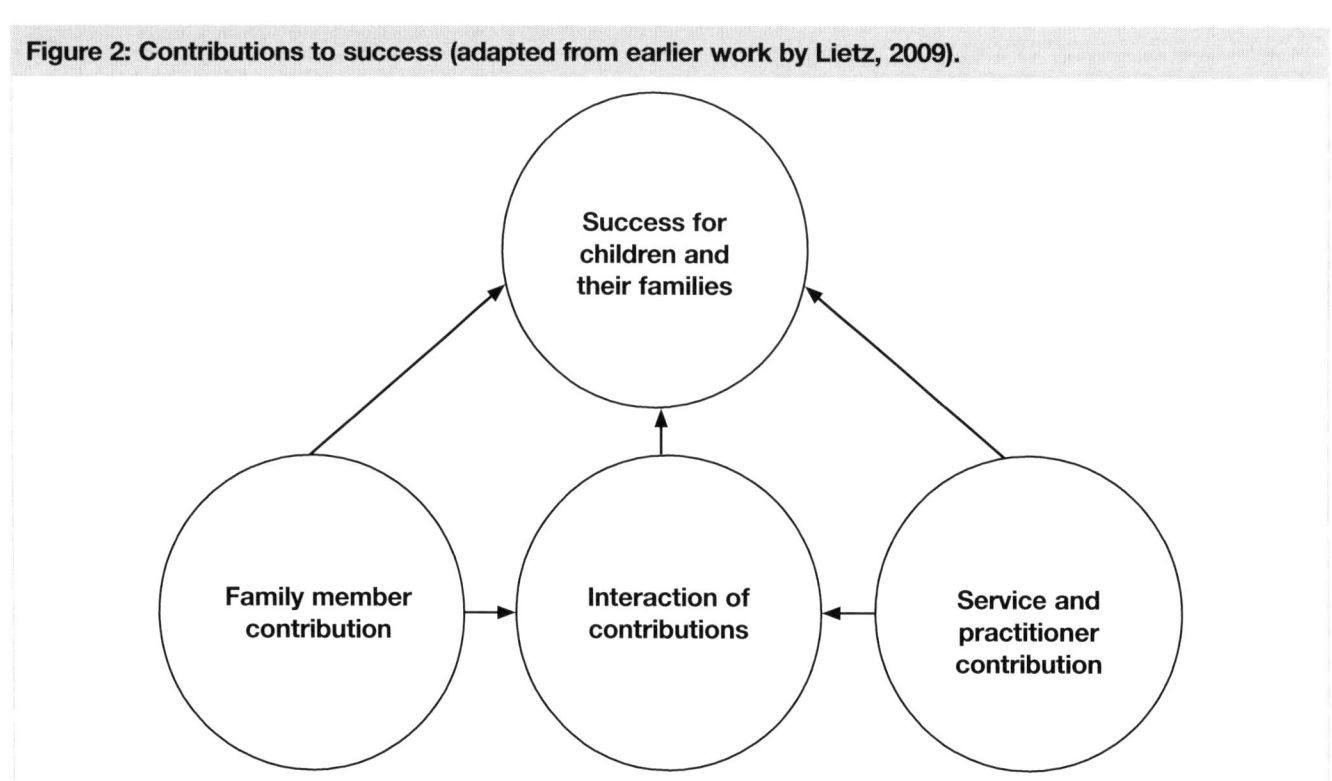

Figure 2: Contributions to success (adapted from earlier work by Lietz, 2009).

The challenges that contemporary safeguarding of children faces is that the search for success is skewed towards the pursuit of externally defined standards; the contribution made by parents and family members to safeguarding their children goes largely unrecognised, and the demands on services at a time of austerity limits opportunities for meaningful relational practice. However, despite these odds, Bluechester provides evidence that the work of parents and practitioners is still creating success stories.

Conclusion

In safeguarding work with children, learning should mean more than acting on the lessons from errors and problematic practice. I have suggested that there are three main areas where success is being established, and in two of these three areas there is potential for family members and practitioners to share their knowledge and wisdom more broadly and for others to learn from it. I do not suggest that this is a straightforward task. Those who create successful outcomes in safeguarding work may be poorly aware of their achievements, may hesitate to reflect on them, or may encounter social barriers to articulating the experience of success. Uncovering and giving attention to success requires leadership, the development of a learning culture, and relationships with children, parents and family members in which they feel their experiences are valued and respected.

It is also important to acknowledge that the success of family preservation in safeguarding situations, emphasised here, is not always possible or preferable. There remain situations where success in its different forms will occur for children while separated from a parent. The concern is, however, that a sense of shared success has been lost in contemporary safeguarding work. It needs definition and legitimation as a prime goal of safeguarding activity.

Finally, I have argued that multiple conceptions of success co-exist in safeguarding work. The challenge for participants is to go beyond the dominant system of evaluating practice, by not only uncovering others' perceptions but also exploring the progress and outcomes from different conceptual standpoints. Services may reach performance targets but parents may find them to be insensitive or inaccessible; practitioners and parents may feel satisfied with intervention but there may be no improvement in measures of the child's development or well-being. A child may be safer as a result of intervention but some participants may harbour a deep sense of injustice about actions undertaken. Critically, exploring the diversity of the way success is experienced – the congruence and the conflicts – permits a deeper understanding of what progress and improvement mean in safeguarding practice.

In order for this sort of understanding to flourish, more systematic change is needed. A change is needed in the way we currently evaluate safeguarding practice. The current system of evaluation is likely to continue to alienate parents and reduce the prospects for meaningful collaboration with families. It focuses more on what organisations do rather than what parents and children experience. We must focus more on achievements and strengths rather than be preoccupied by risk and deficit. We must value shared as well as individual success. Finally, we need to recognise how parents, often in the most difficult of circumstances, successfully safeguard their children, and we need to learn from this.

References

Berg I & Kelly S (2000) *Building Solutions in Child Protective Services*. New York: Norton.

Buckley H, Carr N & Whelan S (2010) Like walking on eggshells: service user views and expectations of the child protection system. *Child & Family Social Work* **16** (1) 101–10.

Dale P (2004) Like a fish in a bowl: parents' perceptions of child protection services. *Child Abuse Review* **13** (2) 137–57.

Featherstone B, White S & Morris K (2014) *Reimagining Child Protection: Towards humane social work with families*. Bristol: Policy Press.

Harris N (1987) Defensive social work. *British Journal of Social Work* **17** (1) 61–9.

HM Government (2015) *Working Together to Safeguard Children: A guide to inter-agency working to safeguard and promote the welfare of children* [online]. Available at: https://www.gov.uk/government/uploads/system/uploads/attachment_data/file/419595/Working_Together_to_Safeguard_Children.pdf (accessed September 2015).

Kemp SP, Marcenko MO, Lyons SJ & Kruzich JM (2014) Strength-based practice and parental engagement in child welfare services: an empirical examination. *Children and Youth Services Review* **47** (1) 27–35.

Lietz CA (2006) Uncovering stories of family resilience: a mixed methods study of resilient families, Part 1. *Families in Society* **87** (4) 575.

Lietz CA (2007) Uncovering stories of family resilience: a mixed methods study of resilient families, part 2. *Families in Society* **88** (1) 147.

Lietz CA (2009) Examining families' perceptions of intensive in-home services: a mixed methods study. *Children and Youth Services Review* **31** (12) 1337–45.

Morgan R (2006) *About Social Workers: A children's views report*. Newcastle: Commission for Social Care Inspection.

Ribner DS & Knei-Paz C (2002) Client's view of a successful helping relationship. *Social Work* **47** (4) 379–87.

Richter KP & Bammer G (2000) A hierarchy of strategies heroin-using mothers employ to reduce harm to their children. *Journal of Substance Abuse Treatment* **19** (4) 403–13.

Saleebey D (2009) *The Strengths Perspective in Social Work Practice*. Boston: Allyn & Bacon.

Schechter C, Sykes I & Rosenfeld J (2008) Learning from success as leverage for school learning: lessons from a national programme in Israel. *International Journal of Leadership in Education* **11** (3) 301–18.

Tilbury C (2004) The influence of performance measurement on child welfare policy and practice. *British Journal of Social Work* **34** (2) 225.

Turnell A & Edwards S (1997) Aspiring to partnership: the signs of safety approach to child protection. *Child Abuse Review* **6** (3) 179–90.

Chapter 17

The Family Model

By Dr Adrian Falkov

This chapter provides a brief summary of The Family Model (TFM) and its use in conjunction with a number of practical tools supporting integrated (family-focused) practice (Falkov, 2012). The six key messages to support family-focused, strengths-based approaches are also included (see www.thefamilymodel.com), together with an example of TFM use in clinical practice (Falkov, 2015).

TFM supports family-focused practice by providing an overarching and comprehensive way of thinking about an individual's needs within their family and social context. It can be used in conjunction with other tools and approaches (for example, the *Continuum of Need* (Falkov, 2014) and the *Family Focused Assessment* (NSW Department of Health, 2010) to facilitate assessment and care planning (Falkov, 2012).

The 'Continuum of Need' approach can help clinicians to map the overall level of a child's needs once they have been identified, which helps clinicians to better define that individual's 'need' within the family context.

The Family Focused Assessment (FFA) provides specific questions and prompts to help clinicians refine types and levels of need and to locate an individual child on the Continuum of Need (Mence & Falkov, 2011). The FFA complements the Continuum of Need by assisting clinicians to define need more accurately by answering the question, 'How will I know what to do?' (once a family has been identified).

Chapter 3 of TFM Handbook (Falkov, 2012) describes in more detail how these tools can be used in conjunction with the Family Model to develop and shape family-focused services for mentally ill parents and their children. While these tools were developed independently of one another, they can be used together within the overarching structure provided by TFM, for a comprehensive, family-focused approach. This process of using both tools together helps to inform care planning and next steps. Where a clinician needs to describe need in greater depth, the Framework for the *Assessment of Children in Need and Their Families* can be incorporated (Department of Health *et al*, 2000).

The Family Model: theoretical underpinnings

TFM formed the key conceptual framework underpinning the *Crossing Bridges* programme (Mayes *et al*, 1998). It provided an understandable, comprehensive and practical way of thinking about the impact of parental mental illness on children and approaches to support family-focused practice. Since then, TFM has undergone considerable revision and enhancement.

Theoretical requirements

A broader approach was required to link the traditional divisions between hospital and community, adult and child, health and social care, protection and prevention. This approach was necessary to tackle one of the unhelpful consequences of specialisation, namely the over-focused and therefore blinkered learning experiences in new generations of students. A shift in learning culture was required, away from exclusive 'single model' approaches to broader (and more sophisticated) approaches better able to integrate health and social sciences.

The biopsychosocial approach was used to represent the complexity of multiple systems in which individuals exist. By drawing on the strengths of biogenetic and psychosocial models (nature via nurture), a more integrated understanding could be facilitated, incorporating mental health, human development, family relationships and parenting.

A systems-informed attitude was also required. Linking the various domains relevant to mentally ill individuals within their family and social context helped to create an approach suitable for staff of varying experience and professional background, working in diverse settings, across different agencies. This approach could incorporate the proximal influences and interactions of an individual within the family, as well as more distal relationships such as neighbourhood and religious networks, as well as schools, cultural and societal values and aspirations.

A developmental (lifespan) perspective was also needed to improve appreciation of the evolving influences and interplay between the developing child and his/her various contexts (such as parenting and the parent-child relationships) over time.

TFM was therefore eclectic and 'non-denominational' in drawing from existing models and providing a broader, more integrated approach.

Key principles

The mental health and well-being of children and adults within families in which an adult carer is mentally ill are intimately linked in at least six ways:

1. Adult/parental mental illness can adversely affect the development, mental health and, in some cases, the safety of children (an adult/parent-to-child influence).

2. Children, particularly those with emotional, behavioural or chronic physical difficulties, can precipitate or exacerbate mental ill-health in their parents/carers (a child-to-parent influence).

3. Growing up with a mentally ill parent can have a negative influence on the quality of that person's adjustment in adulthood, including their transition to parenthood (a childhood-to-adulthood family lifespan influence).
4. Adverse circumstances (such as poverty, lone parenthood, social isolation or stigma) can negatively influence both adult/parent and child mental health (an environment-to-family influence), but resilience means that negative outcomes are not inevitable.
5. The quality of contact/engagement between individuals, families, practitioners and services is a powerful determinant of outcome for all family members (a service-to-family influence).
6. The above five principles and their interactive relationships all occur within a broader social network encompassing cultural and community influences (a broader, more distal, environment-to-family influence).

These principles highlight the key areas and inter-connections between mental illness, parenting and children. They also demonstrate the links over time (childhood-to-adulthood) and across generations. Mental illness has profound implications for the affected individual and for that individual's network of family and social relationships. Given the prevalence of mental illness, major implications ensue, not only for individuals and families, but also for society as a whole.

TFM is a visual illustration of the six key elements ('Domains') involved in understanding how mental illness in a parent/carer can affect their parenting and their children. In turn, children's needs can impact on parents and other family members in various ways. TFM demonstrates the interactions and interdependence between Domains with arrows. It emphasises the reciprocal role of relationships in determining both good and poor outcomes for all family members.

All components must be considered for comprehensive assessment and treatment. The aim of the model is to facilitate an understanding of the processes that underlie and influence how:

➔ Adult/parental mental illness affects children (D1 -> D2).

➔ Mental illness can affect parenting and the parent-child relationship (D1 -> D3).

➔ Parenthood can precipitate and influence mental illness (D3 -> D1).

➔ Children's mental health and developmental needs have an impact on parental mental health (D2 -> D1) and on parenting and the parent-child relationship (D2 -> D3).

➔ Both risk and protective factors interact with parental mental illness, child development and mental health, parenting and the parent-child relationship and with each other in a multi-directional manner (D4 and D1-3 and D4).

➔ Service quality, access and continuity affects identification of families, assessment and intervention and hence influences parental mental illness, child development and mental health, parenting and the parent-child relationship as well as a range of proximal and distal risk and protective factors (including culture and community networks) in a bi/multi-directional manner (D5 and D1-4 and D6).

➔ Cultural and community factors (both proximal and distal environmental influences) interact with parental illness, child development and MH, parenting and the parent-child relationship, and service contacts in a multi-directional manner.

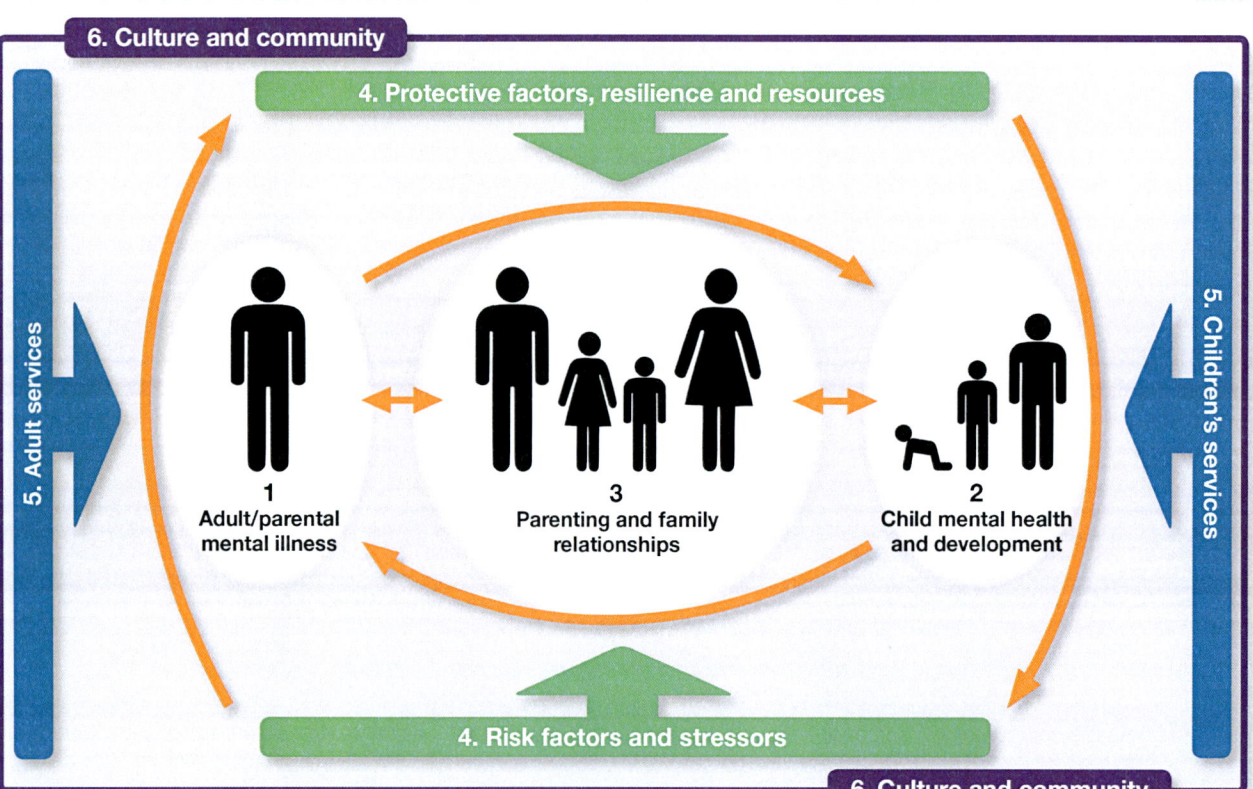

Figure 1: TFM cross-sectional components

(Falkov, 2012)

Figure 2: TFM lifespan and longitudinal perspective

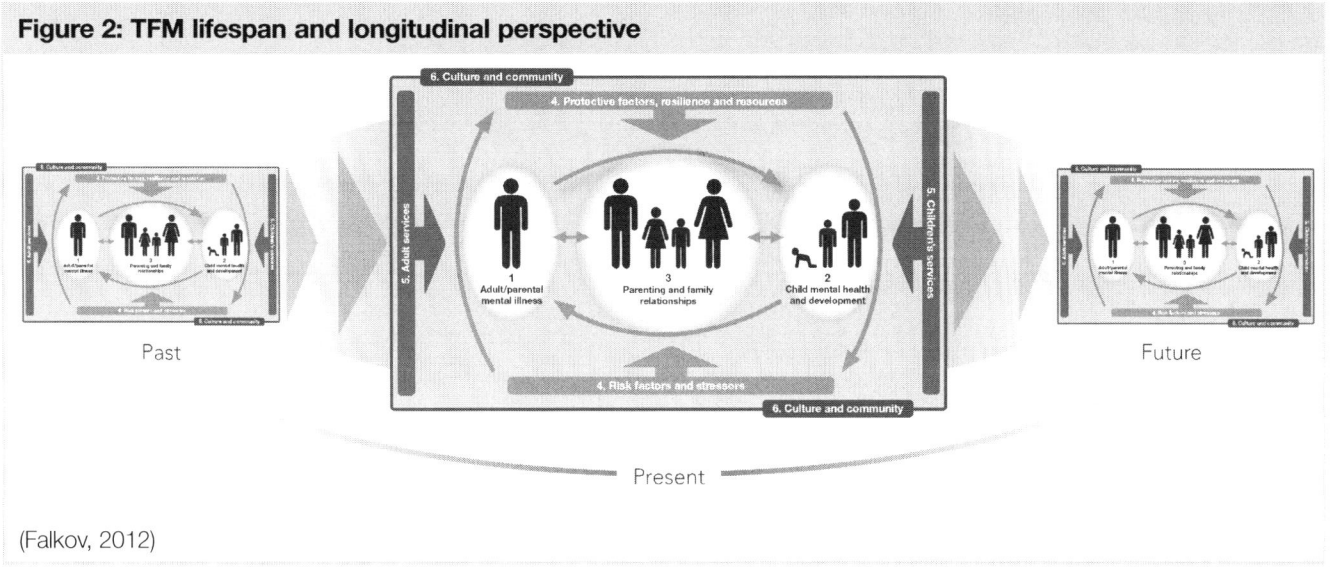

(Falkov, 2012)

How these core components interact with and influence each other determines the quality of an individual's adjustment within his or her family, as well as the adequacy of the whole family's adaptation to living with a mentally ill member.

As well as conveying the relevance of relationships within current family circumstances, TFM also conveys a dynamic perspective of relationship interactions over time (a longitudinal/developmental approach). For example, how multiple factors within and between individuals and their environments interact across the lifespan and between generations. It does this by encouraging thinking about a retrospective ('looking back') and a prospective ('looking forward') approach to practice. Information about need, risk and resilience is used to inform support strategies, treatment plans and recovery. This is based on the evidence linking early adversity with later susceptibility to psychiatric disorder and difficulties in the transition to parenthood – the intergenerational transmission of risk and resilience.

The Family Model: six key messages for family-focused practice

The six overarching principles support six key messages within each of the Domains:

Figure 3: 'Helping parents help children helps parents' (Domain 1)

Adult/parental mental ill-health can affect the development and in some cases the safety of children.

Early identification of parents experiencing mental ill-health and mentally ill adults who are parents/carers is essential for early intervention and prevention measures to reduce risks and promote family mental health.

Figure 4: 'Helping children helps parents help children' (Domain 2)

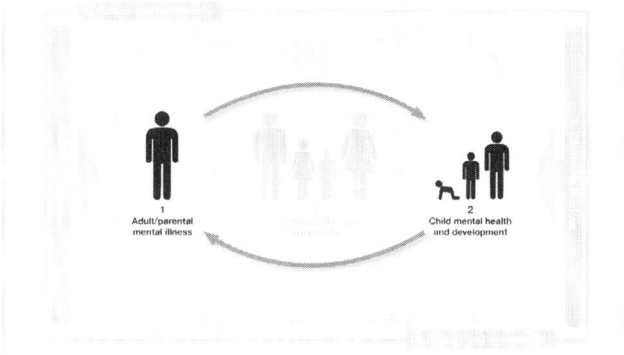

Children, particularly those with emotional, behavioural or chronic physical difficulties, can precipitate or exacerbate mental ill-health in their parents/carers.

Early identification and intervention can reduce the proportion of children and young people whose experience of early adversity (including their own and their parents' mental ill-health) makes them susceptible to later difficulties, including mental ill-health, in their transition to adulthood and parenthood.

Figure 5: 'Good relationships protect' (Domain 3)

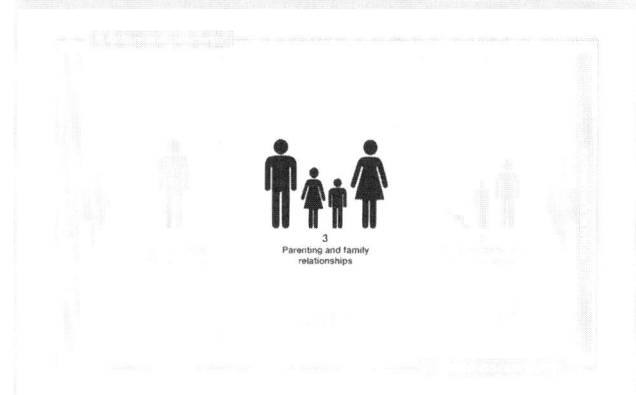

Mental illness can affect parenting and the parent-child relationship, and parenthood can precipitate and influence mental illness.

The links between mental health and parenting thus begin very early in life, are evident across the lifespan and are an important determinant of health and social outcomes in succeeding generations.

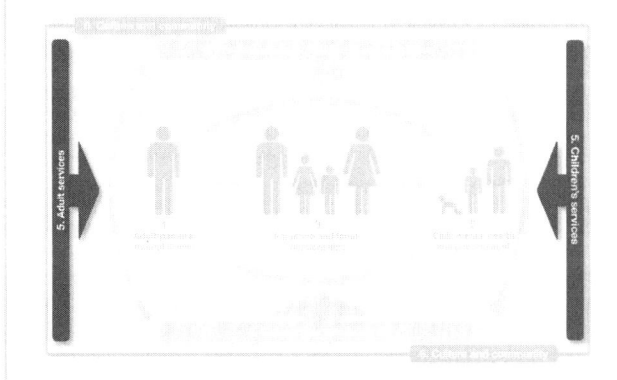

Figure 6: 'Nature via nurture' (Domain 4)

While adverse circumstances (such as poverty, lone parenthood, social isolation and stigma) can negatively influence both child and parental mental health, poor outcomes are not inevitable, effective treatments are available and prevention is possible.

The risks associated with genetic liability for mental illness must be incorporated into the increasing evidence base of effective psychosocial interventions which support recovery, resilience and family mental health.

Figure 7: 'Working better together' (Domain 5)

The quality of contact/engagement between individuals, families, practitioners and services is a powerful determinant of outcome for all family members.

When parents experience mental ill health, they and their children are better supported and protected if agencies and practitioners co-ordinate services and support. Intervening earlier facilitates recovery and has longer term, preventive benefits.

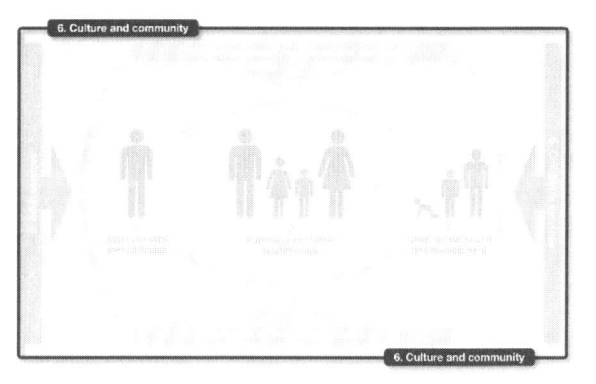

Figure 8: 'Mental health is everyone's responsibility' (D6)

Cultural, community and neighbourhood factors underpin and interact with parental mental ill health, child development and mental health, parenting and the parent-child relationship, and service contacts in a multi-directional, ubiquitous manner.

The quality of social support for individuals experiencing mental illness and their families is an important determinant of the level and type of service need and hence recovery. Tackling stigma is everyone's responsibility.

The Family Model: example of use in clinical practice

Ms M is a 41-year-old English-speaking single mother of Spanish origin who was referred to local mental health centre by her GP for diagnostic review. She had a six-year history of persistent depression for which she had been prescribed at least six antidepressants and was seeing a psychologist. The referral noted that although employed, she was under financial pressure and having to move from her rental apartment. Her daughter, Lizzie, was four-years old.

The clinician undertaking the assessment used TFM diagram to structure thinking about the assessment, analysis of the information and formulating recommendations. In order to better understand maternal experiences and apparent treatment resistance there was a need for additional information about:

→ maternal psychiatric history and background including childhood experiences (D1)

→ child's development and well-being (D2)

→ Ms M's parental role and ways in which depression may have impacted on the parent-child relationship, as well as marital/inter-parental relationship (D3)

→ lifespan and intergenerational vulnerabilities and strengths (D4).

Information from the assessment is summarised below using TFM Domains:

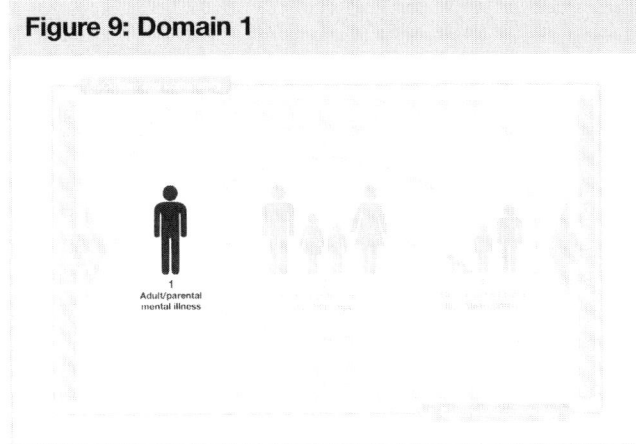

Figure 9: Domain 1

Ms M is a 41-year-old single mother who works part time in an estate agent, with a four-year-old daughter, Lizzie, who recently started preschool.

She described an unhappy, troubled childhood with a two-year history of bulimia in her teens and intermittent social phobia, more troublesome at different points during her life. On looking back, she described being unhappy to the point of depression at about 16 years old, although first diagnosed only six years previously (by a GP). She described having had trials of most of the newer generation antidepressants since the diagnosis was first made, and experiencing partial relief for six to eight months at most, before needing to discontinue each time due to side effects.

She described herself as a perfectionist, able to make friends easily but struggling to sustain them, with a tendency to have unrealistic expectations of others and some degree of rigidity and avoidance, especially during stressful periods.

She was recommencing fluoxetine which had been helpful previously, but at a lower dose than before. She described having a good relationship with her psychologist but was unsure how long she would continue, given that she had already had seven sessions.

Key learning

- Persisting depression – recurrent major depression, partially treated, and complicated by undiagnosed comorbid anxiety disorder and personality traits of perfectionism and psychological rigidity/avoidance.
- Likely to need combination of co-ordinated, integrated multi-modal treatment comprising:
  - review of psychological treatment to ensure evidence-based treatment for depression (e.g. CBT)
  - medication at a dose which delivers best cost-benefit ratio for symptom resolution vs side effects
  - incorporating lifestyle interventions – diet/nutrition, exercise, relaxation and mindfulness and sleep hygiene.
- Discussion with psychologist about ways in which childhood adversities may impact on current functioning including parenting.

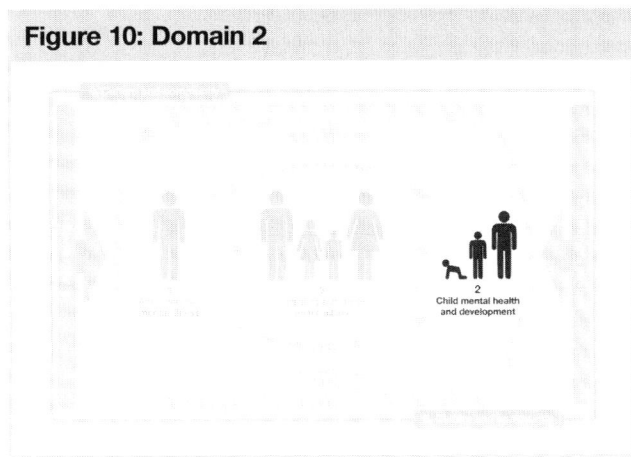

Figure 10: Domain 2

Lizzie was described as 'delightful' and 'my saviour', with an ability to recognise when M was especially stressed. She had struggled initially to separate from M at the start of preschool but had settled and there was a recent report of fighting with one or two of her friends and some fussiness about food, which M had not observed at home. General health was good, no injuries and her immunisations were up to date. The main problem was her poor sleeping pattern for which she had been referred to a paediatrician.

Key learning

- Clarify the quality of the parent-child relationship and the impact of symptoms on child.
- Address sleeping patterns given impact of poor sleep on maternal mood.
- Ensure good communication between (adult and child) professionals.

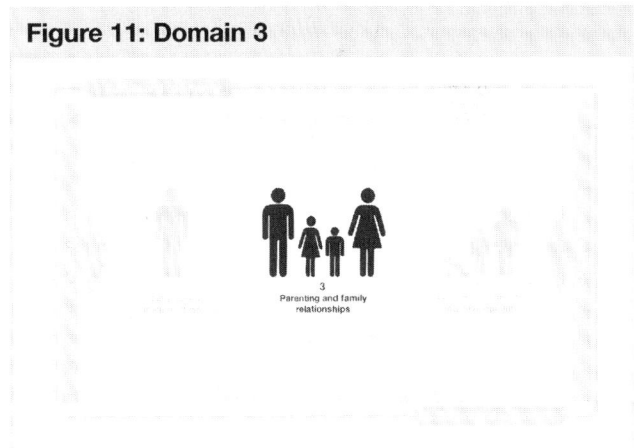

Figure 11: Domain 3

Ms M described doing her best as a parent but feeling guilty about the impact of her symptoms on Lizzie, especially when Lizzie asked why she was sad. Although separated from Lizzie's father due to his gambling and debt problems, she still invited him over to ensure he was able to spend time with Lizzie. She wanted him to be part of Lizzie's life.

Key learning

- Endorse talking with Lizzie about depression so that she has a good understanding of maternal depression, and emphasise that she is not to blame and ensure healthy and appropriate attachment opportunities for Lizzie.
- Ascertain and validate parenting strengths.

→ Ensure good network of support – communicate with school, develop socialisation opportunities.

→ Involve Lizzie's father.

→ Quality of social support for mother (note significant lifespan adversities – D4).

(For more information, see www.copmi.net.au)

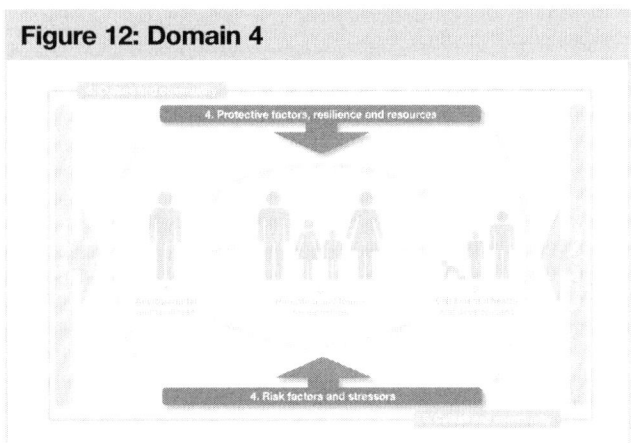

Figure 12: Domain 4

The list of adversities faced by M includes: childhood physical abuse by her father coupled with her mother's inability to protect her, associated emotional maltreatment, abiding sense of confusion and insecurity in childhood, adverse school experiences with bullying, lack of academic and sporting achievements and early exit without good grades, difficult relationship with parents, possible paternal mental illness, intermittent social phobia, difficult intimate partner relationships including divorce and separation from Lizzie's father, and migration to new country in her 20s.

Her strengths include an early interest in and ongoing pursuit of reading, good intelligence and 'psychological mindedness'/ emotional self-awareness, capacity to socialise when well, capacity to persist with tasks and achieve employment/career success, and commitment to doing her best for her daughter.

Key learning

→ Lifespan implications of early adversity and later susceptibility to mental illness and relationship instability.

→ Foster resilience and incorporate strengths into relapse prevention plan:

  → Capacity, through courage, persistence and use of personal assets and strengths to achieve hopefulness, retain compassion and develop a sense of purpose.

  → Good recovery qualities, despite difficult childhood.

  → Commitment to being a good parent and capacity to seek and use help.

→ Consider need for financial advice and assistance with accommodation, if required.

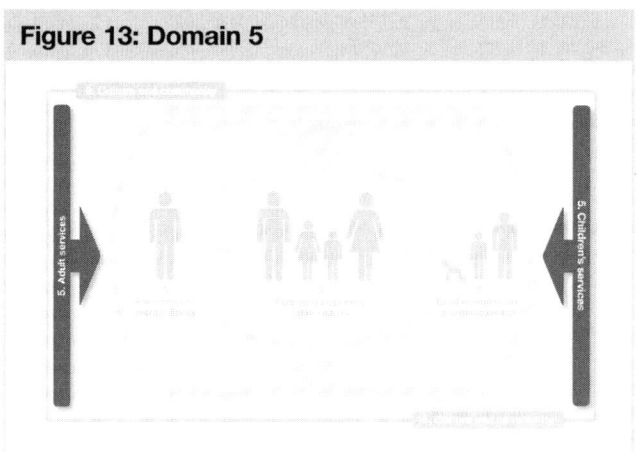

Figure 13: Domain 5

There has been considerable delay in achieving a more comprehensive approach (mental health + parenting + young child's needs) but a good relationship with her GP meant that recommendations were supported, including for ongoing work with a psychologist and referral to a paediatrician to alert about maternal depression.

Key learning

→ Service integration opportunity: primary care (GP) + mental health service with a family focused approached + school + paediatrics.

→ This approach does not add hugely to healthcare costs, especially if, over time, M remains well and Lizzie doesn't experience problems and negative effects (avoiding generational transmission of adversity and illness).

Domain 6

Ms M's Spanish background suggests the need for some inquiry into ways in which she is able to incorporate and impart this aspect of her family story into her and her daughter's life. This highlights the opportunities for local neighbourhood and community support.

Further developments

TFM thus provides a comprehensive framework that illustrates the interactions between a parent's illness, the quality of parenting, the parent/child relationship, the individual attributes and needs of a particular child, and the genetic liabilities, family factors and broader social/community supports that will collectively determine the quality of a child's adjustment at any time point. The interplay between individual, family and environmental vulnerability and resilience will amplify or ameliorate the emergence of any difficulty or disorder over time.

In order to support implementation of family-focused practice, TFM is now being used to develop a (Family Mental Health) module for the Postgraduate Masters in MH course at the University of Oslo/Akersus. Piloting will commence in early 2016. If you are interested in finding out more or participating in evaluating the use of TFM training in different service settings in different countries, please contact the author (adrian.falkov@health.nsw.gov.au).

References

Department of Health, Department for Education and Employment & Home Office (2000) *Framework for the Assessment of Children in Need and Their Families.* London: TSO.

Falkov A (2012) *The Family Model Handbook: An integrated approach to supporting mentally ill parents and their children.* Brighton: Pavilion Publishing.

Falkov A (2014) 'The Continuum of Need', *Gateway to Evidence that Matters*, 17 [Online]. Available at: www.copmi.net.au/research/gems.html (accessed September 2014).

Falkov A (2015) Parental psychiatric disorder: translating The Family Model into practice change. In: A Reupert, D Mayberry, J Nicholson, M Göpfert & MV Seeman (Eds) *Parental Psychiatric Disorder: Distressed parents and their families* (3rd edition). Cambridge: Cambridge University Press.

Mayes K, Diggins M & Falkov A (1998) *Crossing Bridges: Training resources for working with mentally ill parents and their children – Trainer.* Brighton: Pavilion Publishing.

Mence M & Falkov A (2011) *How Will I Know What the Family Needs? The family focused assessment (COPMI) Module: Reference guide for clinicians.* Available from the author: adrian.falkov@swahs.health.nsw.gov.au.

NSW Department of Health (2010) *Policy Directive PD2010_018: Mental Health Clinical Documentation* [online]. Available at: http://www.health.nsw.gov.au/policies/pd/2010/pdf/PD2010_018.pdf (accessed September 2015).

Assessment and interventions

Chapter 18

Emotional neglect, system failure and the Early Years Parenting Unit

By Minna Daum and Dr Duncan McLean

Introduction

Families who emotionally neglect their children are very difficult to help. They are usually unaware of what they are doing and of the impact this has on their children. Neglect is different from trauma in that it is an absence of something rather than an observable behaviour that has an obviously detrimental impact on the child, such as domestic violence or a parent who is exposing their children to behaviour such as drug taking or angry outbursts that are obviously damaging to a child's sense of safety.

Emotional neglect is more insidious, though it can be equally damaging. Social workers and child mental health workers can often be aware that emotional neglect is harmful, but find it difficult to identify and articulate this, as well as to engage families in the seriousness of what is happening. It is our view that only when children's social care can come together with a therapeutic model for helping these families that it is possible to effect any real change. In this paper we will describe a service that has been developed in which the collaboration between children's social care and therapeutic input to the family is combined.

Emotional neglect

Children need to be securely attached to their parents and/or caregivers to develop into adults who can fulfil their potential, manage their feelings, and have co-operative relationships with others. Secure attachment is achieved when caregivers provide not only for the child's physical needs but for their emotional needs as well. Affection, as expressed through both warmth and protectiveness, is essential for a child to develop the basis of any self-esteem, and the sense that they are or could be valued by others. Alongside this is the importance of measured admiration, as the parent takes pleasure in the child's growing sense of competence in all areas of development, from self-care, physical and cognitive abilities, to their developing capacity to become a social being and to take on all the responsibilities that this implies. A lack of admiration leads to an inability in a child to invest in areas of competence, and a stunting of his/her self-esteem. Excessive admiration, meanwhile, can lead to a child having difficulty in overcoming problems, and in recognising vulnerabilities and difficulties in themselves.

A particularly important function of a caregiver is to help their children recognise and manage their own feeling states. This is particularly true of negative feelings such as anxiety, anger, shame and guilt, but is also true to some extent of more positive feelings, such as over-exuberance. Caregivers help children with this in a wide variety of ways. Adults with personality difficulties find this task particularly difficult, as they have experienced poor parenting themselves and have difficulty in both recognising and managing their own feeling states, as well as their children's.

Of particular importance in helping the child recognise their feelings is the caregiver's capacity to mirror these. This is an imaginative process on the part of the caregiver in intuiting a child's state of mind in response to an event and expressing on their face a contained and modified expression of what they imagine the child's state of mind to be. Expressing mild surprise, anxiety, or annoyance will reflect back to the child their own feeling state in a manner that will give them the ability to recognise it for themselves. They will also see a feeling state that is being managed in a calm way, and thereby develop a capacity themselves to manage feelings without being overwhelmed by them. Children who have not experienced adequate mirroring can develop into adults who lack an awareness of various feeling states. They can be anxious or angry with little or no conscious awareness of this; their behaviour, such as avoidance in anxiety or aggressive behaviour when angry, leaves little doubt that they are overcome by feelings, yet if asked about these feelings, they will have little awareness of them.

A further problem that arises out of an individual's difficulty in recognising their feelings is that they will often lack a sense of agency or responsibility in relation to their behaviour, and feel compelled to behave in various ways that they feel they have little or no control over. Much criminal behaviour has this origin.

Other ways in which parents help their children manage their feeling states is by modelling how to do this. Central to a parent's ability to support their children in developing the capacity to recognise and manage their own states of mind is 'mind-mindedness', that is, a capacity to think about the child's developing mind and support their developing capacity to manage various situations that arouse emotions that are potentially overwhelming.

A further means by which a carer supports the containment of difficult feelings is by providing adequate boundaries for the child. These are important not just to keep the child safe, but also to help them develop self-control, in that ultimately they will be able to put boundaries on themselves in relation to impulses that may be unsocial or destructive. Lack of boundaries can be as emotionally neglectful as lack of affection.

System failure

Social workers often recognise elements of emotional neglect, particularly a lack of affection or of boundaries. However, they are often unconfident about evaluating emotional neglect, not so much in terms of lack of affection, but in the parent's failure to help the child both recognise and contain feelings. To evaluate this requires quite close observation of the interaction between parent and child over periods of time, to obtain an understanding of how the carer is imagining the child's mind in a wide variety of circumstances, and thinking about how the child can be helped with these. This can be very difficult to do, especially when a parent is feeling defensive when concerns about their parenting are being raised, which they do not readily understand. Frequently there is a hostile and rejecting attitude on the part of the caregiver, and lacking sufficient evidence to understand how emotionally deprived the child might be, a social worker may withdraw. There may be repeated referrals to social care, with further concerns, though with a similar outcome i.e. withdrawal due to lack of evidence. Later, there may be serious developmental concerns about the child, and guilt in the system over a child being left in a damaging situation, though with little prospect of intervening in an effective way due the age of the child.

Sometimes social care, when faced with a lack of evidence in relation to emotional neglect, will refer to child mental health services. This is frequently unproductive as the carers often fail to engage with these services in any meaningful way. This is extremely frustrating to child mental health services, which will be faced with a family who do not attend, miss appointments, or fail to engage meaningfully with concerns. Often they will complain about social care, and child mental health services may get drawn into colluding with this, feeling that this is the only way to relate to the parents.

Very similar difficulties can arise if social care refers parents to adult mental health services. Carers often remain mistrustful of all services, and are poor engagers, but even if engaging with adult services there is a tendency for the focus to move away from child protection concerns, and that the most pressing reason for the parent to get help is to improve their parenting. In this process, children can continue to be neglected with an erroneous supposition on the part of the system that because the parent is receiving treatment the neglect is being addressed.

The Early Years Parenting Unit

The Early Years Parenting Unit (EYPU) was set up in an attempt to offer a treatment programme to families with a child under five where the parent/s were emotionally neglectful or abusive towards their children as a result of personality difficulties, and that, without intervention, social care were considering removal. It was central to setting up this unit that the service should be an integrated one. There are two essential elements to this integration. First, the therapeutic programme should be fully integrated with children's social care. Second, there would be integration of adult mental health, parenting and child development.

Integration with children's social care

Integration with children's social care (CSC) means that the families are co-managed by both CSC and the therapeutic unit. A referral into the therapeutic unit does not mean that CSC simply withdraws. Co-management means that there is a shared responsibility in relation to child protection, coherent thinking about the aims of intervention and indications of progress or otherwise, and shared decision making. Families are informed that all information will be shared with social care and that there is no confidentiality barrier. The therapeutic unit remains in regular weekly contact with CSC to update them on the progress of the case and to liaise about the progress that the parents and children are making. It is essential that this co-management and co-operation between CSC and the EYPU is maintained throughout, and that the family is aware of this. Without this unified approach, the parents will exploit the relationship with the EYPU to protect themselves from the concerns of CSC, with a tendency to promote a collusive relationship with the therapeutic unit in minimising concerns and vilifying CSC.

This co-working approach is also essential as CSC hold the authority to keep the family in treatment. In effect, they are an important part of the boundary that the therapeutic unit needs to put in place; holding a position that the parents need to change, and that there will be consequences if they do not. Without this authority, the therapeutic input is likely to be impotent, with parents disregarding concerns and refusing to engage, or failing to confront issues as they are too painful.

Integration of adult mental health, parenting and child development

Therapeutic services in relation to failing parents have in the past not offered comprehensive input. Adult mental health services have little expertise in parenting or child development, and will often treat parents' mental health difficulties as if they are separate from their parenting capacity, and often with little thought about how the parents' difficulties are impacting on their children. Though adult mental health services now have a greater awareness than in the past about their child protection duties, this usually extends no further than reporting if they think that a child might be at imminent risk of harm. They often have little awareness of emotional neglect, and will routinely support a parent in resuming their parenting duties while having no evaluation or knowledge about their capacity to be a fully functioning parent.

Child mental health services, though able to focus on parenting and child development, may have little expertise in adult mental health issues, particularly in relation to managing parents with personality difficulties and their emotional dysregulation. Instead of addressing the parents' personality difficulties, clinicians may suggest standard interventions such as parenting courses which these parents are unable to access. Families are often referred back to CSC because they did not engage or make use of what is offered. Sometimes parents will be referred from child to adult services, but there is frequently little co-working between the two and concerns about the child's development are often neglected.

The EYPU was designed to ensure that the three areas of parents' pathology, parenting difficulties and child development were all attended to and related to each other. The therapeutic programme for the EYPU addresses all these areas.

Therapeutic programme

All families that come to the EYPU are cases open to CSC, either as part of the Public Law Outline process, or subject to Child Protection or Child in Need plans. The EYPU worker meets the parent/s in a joint meeting with the social worker to outline the concerns in relation to the parents' ability to parent, with the offer of a therapeutic programme with the explicit understanding that CSC and the therapeutic unit will be working together, and a clear statement of what the consequences will be if the parents fail to engage or change. In subsequent meetings a therapeutic contract is drawn up, outlining the concerns of social care, the parents' goals for change, and the EYPU's expectations in relation to the therapeutic programme.

Engagement in attending the unit is an important and central preliminary task. These families have habitually failed to attend services in the past, and facilitating this process is complex and takes some time. As we have made clear, the authority of social care is necessary in order to spell out the consequences of non-attendance. The unit has to be mindful of the considerable anxieties that parents experience in engaging with professionals. Their lack of trust, their belief in the lack of professional understanding of their difficulties in being a parent both practically and emotionally, their belief that their own needs will be neglected in relation to their role as a parent and their difficulty in engaging in any relationships with others, all need to be acknowledged. One way of thinking about personality difficulties is from the perspective of the parents' difficulties in forming attachment relationships. The unit attempts to establish an attachment relationship between the families and the unit that is experienced as a safe one. This involves giving families practical support in attending, such as providing taxis in the mornings, as well as being very direct with parents about what concerns there are about their parenting and how these are going to be addressed, and showing concern about their individual issues and how the unit will attempt to help them.

The therapeutic programme itself is a three-day per week multi-family programme that families attend for 18 months. It is therefore an intensive and long-term treatment programme, in line with other treatment approaches to people with personality difficulties. Effective interventions with adults with personality difficulties have been shown to require long-term, comprehensive and intensive input if any lasting change is to be achieved. This is in line with the assumption that long-term change is only likely to eventuate through the establishment of a secure attachment relationship between the parents and the therapeutic staff.

The families attend two full days per week (Monday and Wednesday) from 9.30 a.m. – 3.00 p.m. The intervening day is for home visits, assessment meetings, review meetings and supervision of staff. The therapeutic programme involves various elements over the course of the two days. There is multi-family work in which parents are engaged with their children together with other families in various activities such as play, feeding and so on. Therapists work alongside the families both to help them directly and to help them integrate with and support each other in improving their parenting. In addition, there are two adults-only groups per week, while the children are looked after by volunteers. One of the groups focuses on parenting issues, and the other on the parents' individual difficulties. In addition, parents are seen by their key worker for one session a week, either individually or as a couple. There is monitoring and assessment of all aspects of the family's functioning so that the child's development, the parents' capacity to parent, and their ability to manage their own emotional and relational difficulties are all addressed.

The theoretical model for integrating all the different aspects of the family's functioning is that of 'mentalisation'. We cannot give a full explanation of the mentalising stance here, but this can be found in Bateman & Fonagy (2006). In brief, mentalisation can be thought of as the ability to imagine and understand one's own and others' mental states. This is a developmental capacity, and it can be shown that infants of only a few months old are developing a curiosity about the mental states of others. Effective parenting requires a parent to monitor and imagine the mental states of their children, and what they might need help and support with in relation to that. This starts with an ability to gauge a child's physical needs but rapidly this will also come to include the child's emotional needs. Parents with personality difficulties, because they themselves have suffered emotional neglect and/or abuse, have developed very poor capacities to mentalise. For example, they may be unable to imagine that a baby might become distressed in the presence of a shouting adult. Again, a parent may find it very difficult to play with their child as they are unable to enter into the child's imagination.

To help adults who are poor mentalisers, they need a relationship with therapeutic staff in which the staff are constantly curious about the parents' state of mind, and to offer a model of mentalisation by being open and revealing about their own mentalising processes within the therapeutic relationship. In effect, there is a constant process of the therapists questioning parents about what they think is going on either in their own or their child's mind at any particular moment. The therapist also reveals what is going on in his/her mind in response to observing the family. This acts as a model for the mentalising process.

The EYPU has now been running for four years and has been very successful in engaging and working with these very hard-to-engage families. Seventy percent of those families whom the EYPU has attempted to engage have entered the assessment process. Of those, 80% have reached a resolution, either in terms of children being removed into permanent alternative care, or of the parents remaining in treatment and being able to parent their children with little or no social care involvement and improved functioning in both parenting capacity and parental mental health.

Social workers will frequently be in the position of not having a therapeutic team to work with as described above. However, there are some principles that can be drawn from this model that can be utilised when working alone. In assessing a family where there are concerns about emotional neglect, social workers should give themselves an opportunity simply to observe the relationship between parent and child to see how emotional states are expressed and managed. In practice this can be difficult to arrange in the fraught process of assessment, but a request to the parent to just see how they get along with their child in an ordinary way can be made. If concerns are identified these should be communicated to the parent in simple, straightforward and non-technical language.

In relation to the parent, the social worker should attempt to maintain a stance of curiosity about both the parent's way of thinking and the parent's thinking about their child and not get drawn into an oppositional stance in relation to a parent's rigid and defensive thinking. This is extremely difficult but can be developed with practice. Lastly, if a social worker does have a therapeutic team, either child or adult, involved with the family they should attempt to ensure there is proper co-working. This means not just information sharing, but also joint decision making. Services can be resistant to this, but attempting to establish this should be prioritised.

Reference

Bateman A & Fonagy P (2006) *Mentalization-based Treatment for Borderline Personality Disorder*. Oxford: Oxford University Press.

Chapter 19

The Social Work for Better Mental Health adult mental health initiative

Steps towards more effective social work with families with adult mental health problems

By Dr Ruth Allen, Dr Sarah Carr and Dr Karen Linde

This paper reflects on a current and emerging initiative within adult mental health social work in England – Social Work for Better Mental Health (SWfBMH). This aims to support implementation and further develop the propositions within the 2014 source document from the (then) College of Social Work for England, *The Role of the Social Worker in Adult Mental Health Services* (Allen, 2014) which has been promoted by the Chief Social Worker for Adults and the Department of Health.

This 2014 source document was developed after wide consultation within the profession, with social care leaders and with academic social workers. It defined adult mental health social work in terms of five overarching role categories, which are summarised below:

1. Enabling citizens to access the statutory social care and social work services and advice to which they are entitled, discharging the legal duties and promoting the personalised social care ethos of the local authority.

    → Ensuring whole systems of care have cohorts of staff who hold expert knowledge of social care, its ethos and law, and its coherent responsibilities towards people with mental health problems. Staff who can ensure a whole system, integrated response to complex needs (important in this age of fragmentation) and are able to deliver a key part of all organisations' equalities and human rights responsibilities.

2. Promoting recovery and social inclusion with individuals and families.

    → Social workers need to play a full part in interdisciplinary approaches to recovery and social inclusion and need to develop their profession-specific expertise in relation to promoting this. Social workers should be key contributors to breaking down stigma and meeting public duties to ensure people with mental health problems can access ordinary life opportunities. Social workers working across health and social care should be key to integrating recovery approaches and social inclusion within personalisation, and the implementation of the Care Act (2014).

3. Intervening and showing professional leadership and skill in situations characterised by high levels of social, family and interpersonal complexity, risk and ambiguity.

    → Social workers are key to ensuring integrated responses to complexity and risk across systems. Social workers are crucial to complex safeguarding for adults and children and to effective development of family-focused social work in mental health. Practitioners need to be able to balance the rights of different parties and care/control/enablement decision making, and also identify adults and children at risk or in need of support. There should be specific leaders in Mental Capacity Act (2005) practice across systems. 'If not social workers – then who?'

4. Working co-productively and innovatively with local communities to support community capacity, personal and family resilience, earlier intervention and active citizenship.

    → Developing co-production and community skill bases that are needed within the professional mental health workforce. This is key for prevention and promotion of well-being and to meet national policy expectations on mental health and the Care Act (2014). This points to a decidedly 'non-clinical' perspective and foundation for developing an evidence base for social interventions. The longer term strategic public health goals of more mentally healthy communities is a key area for social work innovation.

5. Leading the Approved Mental Health Professional (AMHP) workforce.

    → Ensuring AMHP work is embedded in local authority responsibilities to protect human rights and promote least restriction and independence.

SWfBMH is linked with other national developments attempting to define and frame good social work practice. These include the *Professional Capabilities Framework* for social work (The College of Social Work, 2014) which lays out the expectations of deepening practice throughout the career of all social workers. As practice matures within any sub-specialism there should be an increasing ability to tolerate and work with social risk, ambiguity and complexity, including family complexity. This framework is cross-referenced in detail within the *Role of the Social Worker in Adult Mental Health Services* source document (Allen, 2014).

The five role category definitions for adult mental health social work have been well received across the sector and amongst social workers and social work leaders seeking greater clarity and a chance to 'reclaim' social work identify and focus. This has been lost in many areas, in part as a consequence of the widespread integration of social workers within health-managed provider NHS Trusts since the introduction of statutory powers of delegation within the Health Act (1999) and NHS Act (2006).

While integration of health and social care provision at the point of the experience of the service user and their family is essential, and professional flexibility is undoubtedly required to meet individual needs, good workforce management and effective professional as well as managerial leadership is always required to ensure multi-disciplinarity becomes more, not less, than the sum of its parts in practice.

Since the introduction of the Health Act (1999), statutory mental health services in most parts of England have pursued integrated management of health and social care (and in some cases pooling of commissioning budgets). The predominant model has been of NHS Trusts acting as the hosts of either seconded or transferred social workers and other social care staff. This 'integration experiment' in mental health provides a rich source of learning for future integration initiatives about what conditions do – and do not – give rise to best deployment and development of professional skills and good outcomes for people using services. One thing that has been learnt in adult mental health is how the valuable, professionally distinctive gaze of social work (which the authors define as an intrinsically social, family and systemic perspective) can be lost if organisations hosting multidisciplinary teams are dominated by a limited suite of managerial and 'health' performance targets, and if priorities become focused almost exclusively on the individual service user.

Other professional groups within multidisciplinary services may similarly feel their expertise is not always recognised and developed to their full potential within (what has become in some areas) a 'genericism-led' service system. The difference for social work is, perhaps, its more tenuous position within the NHS workforce. Social work is too often positioned in a difficult, liminal organisational space, managing dilemmas and tensions 'on the ground' which originate in high level strategic ambivalence between local authorities and the NHS.

This uncomfortable and often stressful position is not a solid foundation from which to provide the holistic, multi-factorial, containing and inclusive practice which might be an expectation of mature, confident, systemic social work. It also sets social work in mental health apart from social work colleagues within other parts of adult's services and in children's services, with few opportunities to train or work together other than (often) at points of 'casework' crisis.

The Social Work for Better Mental Health initiative

The SWfBMH initiative in 2015 and 2016 aims to help address the situation described previously through adopting a multi-systemic improvement process for adult mental health social work.

We believe it is one of the first whole-system social work improvement programmes in mental health. It builds on the five role categories work and consists of three resources that support the implementation of clear and effective roles for social workers in adult mental health services. The programme also aims to make the strategic case to commissioners and employers for the development and maintenance of a strong social work workforce across adult mental health – from prevention and early intervention, primary and secondary care and specialist settings. The knowledge and skills described in the role categories are potentially relevant across the whole mental health service landscape.

The three SWfBMH resources are:

1. **The Strategic Statement**
   Aimed at strategic and operational leaders, this document makes the case for further developing social work across mental health, from alignment with primary care and public health within prevention, through to the vital importance of social work knowledge in managing complex, sometimes urgent, social risks.

2. **'How are we doing?'**
   An organisational and workforce self-assessment resource for implementation of the role categories proposed in the source document. This is for integrated health and social care services or social work-only services

3. **'Making the Difference'**
   A framework for direct service user, carer and family feedback and co-production to promote high-quality social work in mental health. It is aimed particularly at social workers and their supervisors, focusing on co-creating practice-based evidence, critical reflection and continuous learning alongside the implementation of evidence-based practice and interventions.

These documents are intended to work as a suite to support organisations and leaders to improve the conditions for great social work practice and outcomes.

The aims of the Social Work for Better Mental Health initiative

Underpinning SWfBMH is attention to promoting and building the evidence base for more relationship-focused practice across adult mental health and a re-balancing towards 'everyday personalisation' within social work encounters. This means making the case for pulling social work back from (often) transactional, multi-professional care co-ordination roles that have emerged out of the primacy of the Care Programme Approach.

Care co-ordination roles have become prone to institutionalised practice around activity measures, rather than outcomes and the lived experience of people using adult mental health services. This can narrow the view of the practitioner and reduce capacity to appreciate and respond to relationships of significance. It also reduces capacity to realise and respond to the needs and capabilities of others in the identified service user's social network, including children and young people. SWfBMH critiques the care co-ordination model for social work deployment.

The implementation of SWfBMH in 2015 and 2016 is proceeding through the identification of 'test sites' (in both the NHS and local authorities) which are being offered facilitated support to understand how they can use the Strategic Statement in their local area; complete 'How are we doing?', the supported self-assessment of the organisational and workforce conditions for social work currently and ambitions for the future, and apply the 'Making the Difference' service user, carer and family feedback tool to help deepen co-production of social work practice.

Building service user, carer and family feedback into routine social work practice

While gaining feedback on practice and experience of services is far from a unique idea, what is distinctive about its 'Making the Difference' framework within SWfBMH is its place within the 'whole system' improvement project, and also its focus on gaining feedback and creating contexts for co-productive dialogue within 'everyday' social work encounters.

Routinely gaining feedback on practice from people we work with is not common within social work, despite this being increasingly embedded in qualifying training (at Batchelor degree and Masters levels), within the Approved and Supported Year in Employment for newly qualified social workers, and within postgraduate Approved Mental Health Professional (AMHP) training. In those specific periods of learning on the social work career journey, students are introduced to the ethical, reflective and educational power of hearing directly how we have or have not impacted and been useful to people we work with. This has been embedded in qualifying training since the social work degree was introduced in 2003. The potential value of co-production of learning and reflective feedback on individual professional practice has been recognised by the Health and Social Care Professionals Council and the relevance of the social work model for other professions is being considered (Beresford, 2014).

Using direct feedback and dialogue with service users may be integral to other specialist post-qualifying training, but, in the absence of a required continuing professional development programme and without a framework of professional social work revalidation requiring direct service user or family feedback, experienced mental health social workers are not required (nor are they requiring of themselves) to regularly hear how their social work practice has been experienced, what its meaning may have been to the person 'in receipt' of the service, and what may have been more effective or welcome.

The contrast between social work educational ideals and the reality of practice and the work environment in mental health seems to be increasing. As Professor Peter Beresford has put it:

'It's beginning to feel as though social work education is actually getting closer to service users and carers than social services organisations are making it possible for practitioners to be. Grassroots reports of ever-increasing bureaucracy, micro-management and paperwork continue, despite the efforts of the social work reform board and Munro inquiries to challenge this....like social work educators (employing organisations)... need to listen to service users, carers and their organisation.' (Beresford, 2014)

SWfBMH is also distinctive in its intention to explore how feedback and co-productive dialogue can be used in routine practice not only with individuals in adult mental health but also with family members of all ages who may be impacted by social work services.

In encouraging the embedding of such feedback from and dialogue with families and social networks as well as individuals, the 'Making the Difference' framework will explore how practitioners recognise the needs and strengths of members of the social system in their own right. This includes the needs of young carers and other young people whom research tells us continue to feel overlooked by mainstream adult mental health practice and, indeed, by some dominant service models.

A framework for testing: an emergent resource

Making the Difference is still developing and will be refined and further developed during 2016 through collaboration with, and feedback from, people using services, carers and families, social workers in practice and academics.

The trial resource that is being tested has two main elements. This first is a tailored questionnaire, using Likert scaling and narrative responses, for use after a social work encounter or intervention (or period of linked interventions) (see Appendix). This has been developed through investigating the evidence for effectiveness of similar questionnaires in the context of professional practice development, and evaluation of competence linked, for instance, to revalidation and appraisal in diverse settings.

However, the evidence base for how such feedback can best be used to contribute to professional development is not well researched in any health or care profession (Chilsolm & Sheldon, 2011) and there is nothing yet at all that is standardised and reliable to evaluate and improve social work practice through feedback.

The evidence that does exist suggests service users often particularly value the quality of relationships, empathy and other interpersonal skills. This provides motivation for further investigation of the social work adage that high-quality social work practice is often distinguishable more by 'how' the work is done, its inclusivity of all involved and the nature of the interaction, rather than strictly by content and technical skill.

Service users and carers have long defined what is important for a positive experience of social worker and social work practice:

> 'They value courtesy and respect, being treated as equals, as individuals, and as people who make their own decisions; they value workers who are experienced, well informed and reliable, able to explain things clearly and without condescension, and who "really listen"; and they value workers who are able to act effectively and make practical things happen… The way workers behave, and what they do or not do, makes a big difference to the way people feel about themselves and the quality of their lives…' (Harding & Beresford, 1996)

Chisolm and Sheldon (2011) also make the point that questionnaires have difficulty capturing the flux, complexity, ambiguity and contradiction of subjective reality. They can *'de-contextualise meaning and distance social action from its natural setting'* (Coyle & Williams, 2000). And they are rarely used with success to gain information about the experiences of people who are most excluded and 'seldom heard'. Chisolm and Sheldon stress elegantly that:

> '….service user feedback is a social rather than technical phenomenon. It is dynamic, bound to contexts and difficult to capture in single snap-shot assessments.' (Chisolm & Sheldon, 2011, p22)

This points to the second aspect of Making the Difference, which is developing and field testing a framework for social workers and the people they work with. A framework to engage in meaningful dialogue to explore the situated experience of receiving social work support and intervention, and what would have made it more effective.

Setting the conditions for this is complex and requires consideration of the service user, carer or family's experience and expectations of power and safety to speak. In addition, we also need to consider the practitioner's concerns of exposure and how feedback and the content of discussions may be used if there is a link to, for instance, supervision or appraisal. There are, of course, existing frameworks for holding such dialogues with adults and children (e.g. the GEMS framework which uses a solution focused approach to encourage creative dialogue). However, the intention of Making the Difference is to co-produce a framework that is tailored to the context of mental health practice.

The SWfBMH project group is thus co-developing a field test framework with social work practitioners, supervisors and people who have used services, carers and family members. This will include young carers and children.

Future research and implementation

After being initially commissioned by the Department of Health, SWfBMH is currently funded only through its consultation offer to organisations wishing to implement all or some of the resources. This is an ongoing offer for any organisation providing or commissioning mental health services.

The medium-term aim is to take the findings from the field test activities in 2015 and 2016 and treat these as a 'feasibility study' for further funded research into the application of the organisational development resource 'How are we doing?' and Making the Difference. In relation to the latter, through this process we hope to identify how social work in mental health can routinely turn ongoing feedback and dialogue about social work practice into ongoing development both of individual practitioners and whole workforces. Through this we hope ensure the process is useful and rewarding for those using social work services. Indeed, in the true spirit of co-production, if done properly, this is a real opportunity for service users and families to have a strong sense of contribution to service improvement and empowerment over the discourse of practice and what is important.

Through this we hope to test how we can 'make the difference' to people using services, their children, partners and family members through developing greater curiosity, openness and willingness to change mental health social work practice in light of feedback and co-productive conversations.

References

Allen R (2014) *The Role of the Social Worker in Adult Mental Health Services.* London: The College of Social Work.

Beresford P (2014) Social work education leads the way on involving service users and carers. *The Guardian* 3 June.

Chilsolm A & Sheldon H (2011) *Service User Feedback Tools. An evidence review and Delphi consultation for the Health Professions Council.* Oxford: Picker Institute Europe.

Coyle J & Williams B (2000) An exploration of the epistemological intricacies of using qualitative data to develop a quantitative measure of user views of health care. *Journal of Advanced Nursing* **31** (5) 1235-1243.

Harding T & Beresford P (1996) *The Standards We Expect – What service users and carers want from social services workers.* London: National Institute for Social Work.

The College of Social Work (2014) *The Professional Capabilities Framework* [online]. The British Association of Social Work. Available at: https://www.basw.co.uk/resource/?id=1137 (accessed September 2015).

Appendix

Proposed 'Making the Difference' questionnaire
Field test version, September 2015

Proposed core service user and carer feedback questions

These questions have been revised in response to the feedback from senior mental health social work leaders. They now represent a combination of what social work leaders, service users and carers regard as important for social work practice. Specific questions have been modified to capture the unique contributions of social work to mental health.

Questions to be rated on a 5-point scale:

Cluster to assess knowledge, professionalism, co-production
- → The social worker always explained things clearly and kept me informed about what was happening.
- → The social worker explained to me what my rights were.
- → The social worker went away and looked at all the options and was open and honest with me about what they were.
- → The social worker made sure I had enough information and advice to make my own decisions.
- → I could ask questions and the social worker was able to answer them properly.
- → The social worker knew about things going on in my neighbourhood that I would enjoy or find helpful.

Cluster to assess professionalism
- → The social worker was polite and treated me with respect.
- → The social worker came on time or let me know if they were running late.
- → The social worker was easy to contact.
- → The social worker did what they said they would do.

Cluster to assess professionalism, values, diversity, intervention and skills, co-production
- → I felt comfortable talking to the social worker.
- → I felt the social worker understood what I was saying and how I was feeling.
- → I felt the social worker understood my whole situation and the things going on in my life.
- → I felt the social worker was trustworthy and reliable.
- → The social worker asked about and showed respect for my background and culture.
- → The social worker built on my ideas and experiences when we were making decisions.

Cluster to assess values and ethics, intervention and skills, knowledge, contexts and organisations
- → The social worker gave me time and space to tell my own story in my own way.
- → The social worker was interested in me as a whole person, not just my mental health problem.
- → The social worker wanted to know about my family, friends or neighbours.
- → The social worker talked openly with me about taking risks and staying safe, and took my experiences and opinions seriously.
- → The social worker wanted to know what I was good at and what I enjoyed doing.

Cluster to assess intervention and skills, knowledge, co-production
- ➔ The social worker helped me take control of things.
- ➔ The social worker and I worked as equals to draw up a plan.
- ➔ The social worker made practical things happen that helped me.

Free text questions:
- ➔ What do you think the social worker did well?
- ➔ What do you think the social worker could have done differently?
- ➔ How has the social worker made a difference to you?
- ➔ Could anyone else have done what the social worker did?
- ➔ Are there any other things you'd like to say about your social worker?

Working together

Chapter 20

Co-work: working in pairs enables effective whole family sessions

By Dr Frank Burbach

Despite increasing interest in whole-family interventions, little attention has been paid to how family sessions should be facilitated. This paper describes various ways of facilitating family sessions and sets out the arguments for involving two (or more) clinicians. The case for co-work is made, including: continuity of support, consistent messages, supervision and support, attending to multiple voices, reflective conversations and collaborative therapeutic practice. It argues that the importance of a stable therapeutic relationship is paramount and that this provides sufficient justification for any small increase in staff costs. In addition, it argues that the quality of the therapeutic intervention is significantly enhanced if co-therapy is employed.

Introduction

It is increasingly being recognised that mental health problems have a significant impact on parenting, the parent-child relationship and the child. It is also recognised that adult and children's services need to develop joined up approaches. As a result, there is increasing interest in delivering whole-family interventions, both in the various 'troubled families' initiatives and in mental health services (Morris et al, 2008). There is growing evidence of their effectiveness (Carr, 2009a; 2009b; Crane, 2008; DCLG, 2012; Stratton, 2011) but a key aspect of practice has received relatively little attention to date.

This issue of co-working is seldom discussed in the literature and has not been researched to any significant extent. An exception is the study of co-therapy as a training method in which, for example, Hendrix et al (2001) found that it was a useful training method, although different co-therapy combinations did not affect outcomes. Positive aspects associated with co-therapy were reported as a greater willingness to take risks, finding their colleague's perspective on the case useful (as well as their strengths, expertise and knowledge) and being able to comment on the process of the session as an intervention.

Within family intervention in psychosis, it is common practice to use a co-therapy model and it is strongly recommended by some of the originators of the field (e.g. Kuipers et al, 2002), but there is an ongoing debate about employing more than one therapist. Another common psycho-educational family intervention approach, Behavioural Family Therapy for psychosis, is usually provided by a single family worker, partly because family sessions are easier to arrange but primarily for reasons of cost. Co-therapy is commonly used in couple therapy, with the ideal pairing being a male and a female therapist (if working with a heterosexual couple). Systemic family therapy is often provided by pairs or teams of therapists in NHS mental health services, but usually by one therapist if they are in private practice. Most of the published considerations of 'co-therapy' are to be found in the older systemic couple and family therapy literatures (e.g. Walrond-Skinner, 1976; Treacher & Carpenter, 1984).

Co-work does not appear to have been considered in the literature on 'troubled family' support programmes. Many of these intensive, multi-professional and multi-agency family support programmes are delivered by a single worker who provides wide ranging support to 'multi-problem' families. These workers liaise closely with professionals from a wide range of services, and sometimes accompany family members to appointments with other agencies, but rarely involve them in actual family sessions. An exception is the Westminster Family Recovery Project (FRP) (Thoburn, 2015), where the day-to-day work with the family is shared by two lead professionals – the FRP intensive outreach worker and the lead worker for the children (usually a social worker). The specialist worker sometimes acts as a consultant to the outreach worker and at other times they work jointly.

The importance of the therapeutic relationship

'Multi-problem' families typically report feeling increasingly powerless as more and more experts get involved. The success of intensive family support programmes appears to be related to the stable bond formed with the worker who takes on the role of 'buffer', or 'filter', between the family and the often large number of agencies involved. Services such as Wandsworth's FRP, a multi-agency service set up by Wandsworth Council, and a wide range of statutory and voluntary sector agencies including the police, health services and Job Centre Plus, aim to create an intensive team around the family (Jones et al, 2015) without confusing or overwhelming them. In this project, the traditional network of ever-increasing helping agencies around the family is replaced with a 'network around the professional' – where the network's role is to support the key professional who is able to create a strong yet flexible therapeutic relationship with the family.

Psycho-therapeutic models, in particular Bowlby's attachment theory (Bowlby, 2008), provide a clear theoretical rational for the provision of a secure attachment bond to the worker. Feeling safe and secure (a 'secure base') enables people to be less anxious and defensive, and frees up their ability to creatively solve problems and take small positive steps into the unknown. In contrast to the stress of relating to a range of concerned professionals, in FRPs family members report forming more trusting relationships with their intensive outreach worker and feel that they can depend on him/her. A family worker typically advocates on their behalf, supports them to solve practical problems, provides emotional support, and generally focuses on their strengths. In Wandsworth, positive outcomes such as a reduction in depression, increased training, education and employment, and more consistent parenting and boundary setting were achieved. This appeared to be related to an effective therapeutic relationship with the family members, who reported that the involvement of the FRP was much more intensive, and much more demanding, than they had experienced before or had expected (Jones et al, 2015).

Some clinicians (e.g. Aggett, 2012; Summer, 2015) have given a great deal of thought to the type of therapeutic relationship that enables such outcomes. They advocate a 'permission seeking' ethical stance and clinical practice that address the power imbalances often impeding engagement with socially marginalised families. Family therapists working with marginalised client groups have also described adopting co-therapy 'live supervision/reflection' or in-the-room reflecting teams (Anderson, 1991) to counter the disempowering effects of the traditional family therapy observing team of supervisors. For example, Smith and Kingston (1980) consulted to each other with the family present in a probation setting and Vetere and Cooper (2001) describe this in the context of working with violence in families.

Many UK children and families social care services have adopted the Reclaiming Social Work model (Goodman et al, 2011) in order to connect with 'hard-to-reach' families. Services to these families are provided by small teams whose practice is underpinned by a systemic family therapy model. These 'units', or 'pods', are led by a consultant social worker who is the case holder and also manages and supervises the other members of the unit. The composition of these units varies, but often include two or three other clinical staff (another social worker, family therapist, children's worker) and an administrator. Jenny Summer's article (2015) describes a home-based live-supervision group that has been successfully used in Cambridgeshire to engage with socially marginalised families and enhance the clinical skills of her colleagues in the child in need unit that she leads.

These various service examples indicate a basic awareness of the importance of the therapeutic relationship, the need for continuity and the creation of a 'safe therapeutic space'. There are various ways of achieving this, and to my knowledge there has not been any research comparing models. Drawing on our practice in Somerset with families where a member has psychosis (Burbach, 2015), I propose that employing a co-therapy approach at the heart of the therapeutic endeavour is particularly beneficial and the main advantages are outlined below.

The case for co-work

1. Continuity of support

Although having a professional who provides stable, ongoing support is crucial to enable positive change, there is a danger of 'putting all the eggs in one basket'. Many people in troubled families have repeatedly experienced being let down by significant others (parents, professionals etc.) and may react particularly badly if their worker becomes unavailable due to illness, change of job or any other factors. The chances of this occurring can be minimised by utilising two clinicians. These pragmatic considerations are the first reason for recommending creating a relationship between at least two professionals and any 'troubled family'. Similarly, in assertive outreach mental health services, a team approach is employed to engage with their high risk, 'revolving door' clients. This approach enables clients to form long-term therapeutic relationships with three or more people so that continuity of support is ensured seven days a week. Continuity is also enabled in formal family therapy sessions – these can go ahead even if a therapist is unexpectedly unavailable, since a co-therapist or team member can take over and facilitate the session rather than having to rearrange the appointment.

2. Consistent messages

Co-working is particularly helpful when different agencies are involved. In such cases, we recommend having a worker from each main agency forming a stable co-working pair as this reduces the likelihood of family members receiving mixed messages. For example, where different members of the family are referred separately to child and adult mental health services, it is helpful to offer family sessions with a clinician from each service. A co-work pair comprising one person from the statutory and one from the non-statutory services is another good example. Ideally, these inter-agency co-working arrangements can be built in to the service model. Gloucestershire Young Carers' InterAct project, for example, provides family sessions where the programme facilitator maintains contact with the parent's care co-ordinator throughout. The care co-ordinator then attends the final session.

3. Supervision and support

Another advantage of working in pairs is that it enables mutual support and 'live supervision'. Sessions with families can often be challenging due to the complexity of the issues being presented, and having two therapists means that sessions are less likely to get 'stuck' as each of them will be able to offer their knowledge, skills and experience. The two workers can also share responsibilities and workload (e.g. follow-up administrative tasks), which prevents worker overload and burnout.

In family sessions it can also be difficult for a single worker to attend to the needs of everyone present and to respond to the range of verbal and non-verbal simultaneous communications. Family therapists often recommend that one therapist takes the lead and that the other therapist(s) take an 'observer position' and comment on the process where appropriate. The lead clinician may not have noticed that a member of the family has shed a tear or fallen silent at a particular point in the session. Noticing this can ensure that such issues are addressed and that everyone feels included and attended to. The observer co-therapist may also notice information that has been presented but overlooked due to the rate or complexity of the conversation.

An advantage of the co-therapy model is thus, in part, that it is like having a supervisor in the room. While one therapist is engaged in talking with the family, the other is able to observe the process and intervene where appropriate. The co-therapist can help to keep the therapy on track, introduce new ideas and help their colleague should they feel 'stuck'. The 'observer co-therapist' can also intervene and interrupt the process when the session is becoming unhelpful. A comment or question may be sufficient but occasionally a more forceful interruption may be required, for example when family members get stuck in an excessively critical interactional pattern or are becoming overtly abusive.

At times during the meeting it may be helpful for the therapists to have a brief reflective conversation with one other, in which they may comment on the way in which the meeting has progressed and discuss options for the rest of the session or share observations and tentatively offer alternative perspectives. It is an unusual experience for families to hear themselves being talked about and this can effectively interrupt unhelpful interactions as they stop to listen. In addition, families value these opportunities to reflect upon themselves and consider new perspectives (see '5. Attending to multiple voices, reflective conversations and collaborative therapeutic practice').

The idea that 'many heads are better than one' especially applies to the most challenging issues that can arise. Many dilemmas are complex, without there being a right or wrong response, and it is in such situations that it is particularly useful to be able to 'bounce ideas' around with a co-worker, both in the session and afterwards. Although post-family session 'debriefing' and support may be available from a supervisor, many therapists value having this reflective conversation with a co-worker who has experienced the session and, arguably, may have a more accurate perception of the issues.

It is also increasingly recognised that co-workers, by sharing responsibility, are generally able to take more positive risks and are less likely to make 'knee jerk' responses.

4. Modelling

Modelling (i.e. learning by observing the co-therapists) is an advantage of co-work emphasised in the earlier behavioural and psychodynamic literature on co-therapy. This process is undoubtedly effective in some cases, but families are not necessarily going to copy the more effective communication and positive relationship of the therapists. In addition, an uneven co-therapy relationship, or one which mimics unhelpful relationships in the family (e.g. a dominant male therapist and a passive female therapist) may unwittingly reinforce unhelpful relational patterns (Dowling, 1979).

In psycho-educational/behavioural family intervention approaches for psychosis, the two therapists may well find it helpful to demonstrate a particular communication or problem solving technique, but again this could also have the unintended effect of disempowering the family as they critically compare their own skills to those demonstrated, and it could be argued that any demonstration of new skills should rather be done by a therapist working with a family member, or by family members role-playing the desired skill (Barker & Chang, 2013).

In certain types of therapy, therefore, the modelling process may not be particularly helpful. On balance, however, I would agree with Lax (1995) that the reflecting conversations (see '5. Attending to multiple voices, reflective conversations and collaborative therapeutic practice') that are a feature of contemporary co-therapy inherently provide an opportunity for modelling a helpful style of communication. What family members will observe is therapists considering a multiplicity of ideas, carefully listening to each other's views, and offering, and sometimes opposing, ideas in a tentative, positive and respectful manner. As this is done without an expectation that the family members emulate this, it does not run the risk of disempowering family members (although some family members may think that this is rather odd 'therapist talk'!).

5. Attending to multiple voices, reflective conversations and collaborative therapeutic practice

Co-work also enables the more collaborative, reflective practice associated with socio-constructive systemic therapy approaches. It enables the creation of richer, more elaborated meanings similar to the reflecting team approach (Andersen, 1991) or the dialogic approaches (Bertrando, 2007; Seikkula & Arnkil, 2014). These approaches recognise that people are more likely to find their own solutions if they are encouraged to voice their experiences and develop their own understandings, and reflective conversations appear to be an effective way of facilitating this process. These reflective conversations are not instructive or directive in nature, but are conducted in a tentative manner, where a range of ideas is offered for the family to consider, comment on and incorporate where they seem appropriate. These conversations need to be brief, genuine and positive in nature, use language that is easily understood by the family, emphasise solutions rather than problems, and be respectful and valuing of the family. These conversations can be highly effective if conducted sensitively (Andersen, 1995; Lax, 1995; Williams & Auburn, 2015), but this approach does not suit all families (Jenkins, 1996) and it is important to seek the family's feedback as to its value.

The impressive outcomes achieved by the Open Dialogue mental health services in Western Lapland, Finland (Seikkula et al, 2006), is ascribed to their dialogic approach and encouraging 'polyphony'. In these 'network' sessions two or three therapists attend to and value the 'multiple voices' in the room, not only the people present at the sessions but also the 'internal voices' that each person carries with them (e.g. the 'voices' of their father, mother, friends etc.). This approach contrasts with the 'certainties', or 'narrow descriptions' that are delivered in psycho-educational approaches. Co-therapists who genuinely value multiple descriptions and participate in family sessions in a genuine, authentic manner facilitate the deepening of the therapeutic relationship.

The use of reflective conversations in a co-therapy approach does not appear to have been specifically investigated as yet, but the ability of co-therapists to create an enabling therapeutic relationship with family members has been supported by a number of studies conducted with the family intervention for psychosis service in Somerset. Participants in our first research study evaluating the service said they valued, *'Open discussion in a safe and supportive environment'* and appreciated the collaborative process:

> 'It felt as if we had the first say and they (therapists) would follow what we wanted, but they might come up with suggestions as well, but it felt as if our needs came first.'

This was often a profound experience:

> 'I felt very much understood. That was very overwhelming in a way, having come from a place where we weren't understanding each other at home, to have two people who were empathetic there for me and for our son.'

The family sessions were therefore experienced as a lifeline:

> 'Without the help I don't think we'd have been in business. I don't think we'd have been able to carry on normally.' (Burbach & Stanbridge, 2009; Stanbridge & Burbach, 2007; Stanbridge et al, 2003)

In more recent qualitative research studies (Allen *et al*, 2013; Rapsey *et al*, 2015), the ability of the co-therapists to create a safe therapeutic space – 'a different world' – was again highlighted. Family sessions provided the opportunity for family members to tell their own story and become more aware of each other's experiences. This seemed influential in developing a sense of agency and was described as 'healing'. One participant reported:

> 'Each of us would have come in originally with totally different perceptions of what the issues were and how we reacted to them in the past, and we found that by sharing those experiences we realised we had differences and we had a much better common understanding at the end of it.' (p10)

Another person described how understanding the *'different perceptions … dissipates the problem'* (Rapsey *et al*, 2015, p11).

The following quotes give more specific feedback on the co-therapy aspect of the service:

> 'Because there was two people coming, they saw different sides as well, so they bounced ideas off each other and so it just widened and widened and you began to think again, oh I didn't think of it that way.' (p112)

> 'Yeah, having two facilitate the actual session was brilliant and the two professionals cos say we were discussing something I don't understand from my side or my parent's didn't understand.' [sic] (p113)

> 'The other therapist has been very good when it comes to knowing more about the medical sort of stuff, the drugs and people.' (p128)

(Rapsey, 2012)

Conclusion

Although there is increasing recognition of the importance of a stable therapeutic relationship, services are under constant pressure to use resources more efficiently. It will always be a dilemma as to how to deploy clinical staff in the most clinically effective and efficient manner, but the creation of a strong therapeutic relationship with two co-workers appears to be a very sensible option. Having two workers rather than one involved in regular therapeutic meetings with families will result in a small increase in staff costs, but these will be offset by preventing the greater costs associated with the almost inevitable breakdown of some of the therapeutic relationships with single workers.

Resilience and sustainability of the therapeutic relationship is not the only advantage of co-therapy models, however. The other reasons to adopt this approach all contribute to improved quality of the work with families. In particular, the more sophisticated collaborative therapeutic practice enabled by reflective co-therapy can reasonably be expected to improve outcomes and therefore achieve broader savings. This is a testable proposition and it is hoped that this will be researched in a range of clinical settings.

References

Aggett P (2012) Responsiveness, permission-seeking and risk: three motifs in the development of outreach family therapy services and therapist self-reflexivity. *Context* **120** 6–9.

Allen J, Burbach FR & Reibstein J (2013) 'A different world': individuals' experience of an integrated family intervention for psychosis and its contribution to recovery. *Psychology and Psychotherapy: Theory, Research and Practice* **86** (2) 212–228.

Andersen T (1991) *The Reflecting Team: Dialogues and dialogues about the dialogues*. New York: Norton.

Andersen T (1995) Reflecting processes; acts of informing and forming: You can borrow my eyes, but you must not take them away from me! In: S Friedman (Ed.) *The Reflecting Team in Action: Collaborative practice in family therapy* (pp11–37). New York: Guilford Press.

Barker P & Chang J (2013) *Basic Family Therapy*. Chichester: Wiley-Blackwell.

Bertrando P (2007) *The Dialogical Therapist: Dialogue in systemic practice*. Karnac Books.

Bowlby J (2008) *A Secure Base: Parent-child attachment and healthy human development*. Basic Books.

Burbach FR (2015) Brief family interventions in psychosis: a collaborative, resource-oriented approach to working with families and wider support networks. In: B Pradhan, N Pinninti & S Rathod (Eds) *Brief Interventions for Psychosis: A clinical compendium*. Springer (forthcoming).

Burbach FR & Stanbridge RI (2009) Setting up a family interventions service. In: Lobban F & Barrowclough C (Eds). Chichester: Wiley-Blackwell.

Carr A (2009a) The effectiveness of family therapy and systemic interventions for child-focused problems. *Journal of Family Therapy* **31** (1) 3–45.

Carr A (2009b) The effectiveness of family therapy and systemic interventions for adult-focused problems. *Journal of Family Therapy* **31** (1) 46–74.

Crane RD (2008) The cost-effectiveness of family therapy: a summary and progress report. *Journal of Family Therapy* **30** (4) 399–410.

DCLG (2012) *Working with Troubled Families: A guide to the evidence and good practice.* London: Department of Communities and Local Government.

Dowling E (1979) Co-therapy: A clinical researcher's view. In: S Walrond-Skinner (Ed) *Family and Marital Psychotherapy: A critical approach.* London: Routledge & Kegan Paul.

Goodman S, Trowler I & Munro E (2011) *Social Work Reclaimed: Innovative frameworks for child and family social work practice.* London: Jessica Kingsley.

Hendrix CC, Fournier DG & Briggs K (2001) Impact of co-therapy teams on client outcomes and therapist training in marriage and family therapy. *Contemporary Family Therapy* **23** (1) 63–82.

Jenkins D (1996) A reflecting team approach to family therapy: a delphi study. *Journal of Marital and Family Therapy* **22** 219–238.

Jones R, Matczak A, Davis K & Byford I (2015) 'Troubled Families': A team around the family. In: K Davies (Ed) *Social Work with Troubled Families: A critical introduction* (pp124–158). London: Jessica Kingsley.

Kuipers L, Leff J & Lam D (2002) *Family Work for Schizophrenia: A practical guide.* London: Gaskell.

Lax WD (1995) Offering reflections: Some theoretical and practical considerations. In: S Friedman (Ed) *The Reflecting Team in Action: Collaborative practice in family therapy* (pp145–166). New York: Guilford Press.

Morris K, Hughes N, Clarke H, Tew J, Mason P, Galvani S, Lewis A, Loveless L, Becker P & Burford G (2008) *Think Family: A literature review of whole family approaches.* Social Exclusion Task Force, Cabinet Office.

Rapsey EHS (2012) *Exploring the Process of Family Interventions in Relation to Attachment, Attributions and the Maintenance of Difficulties. An IPA study* [online]. Exeter: University of Exeter. Available at: https://ore.exeter.ac.uk/repository/handle/10036/3681 (accessed September 2015).

Rapsey EHS, Burbach FR & Reibstein J (2015) Exploring the process of family interventions for psychosis in relation to attachment, attributions and problem maintaining cycles. An IPA study. *Journal of Family Therapy* DOI: 10.1111/1467-6427.12085

Seikkula J, Aaltonen J, Alakare B, Haarakangas K, Keranen J & Lehtinen K (2006) Five-year experience of first-episode nonaffective psychosis in open-dialogue approach: treatment principles, follow-up outcomes, and two case studies. *Psychotherapy Research* **16** 214–228.

Seikkula J & Arnkil TE (2014) *Open Dialogues and Anticipations: Respecting otherness in the present moment.* Tampere: National Institute for Health and Welfare.

Smith D & Kingston P (1980) Live supervision without a one-way screen. *Journal of Family Therapy* **2** (3) 379–387.

Stanbridge RI & Burbach FR (2007) Involving carers (Part 1). In: Froggatt D, Fadden G, Johnson DL, Leggatt M & Shankar R (Eds) *Families as Partners in Mental Health Care: A guidebook for implementing family work.* Toronto: World Fellowship for Schizophrenia and Allied Disorders.

Stanbridge RI, Burbach FR, Lucas A & Carter K (2003) A study of families' satisfaction with a family interventions in psychosis service in Somerset. *Journal of Family Therapy* **25** 179–202.

Stratton P (2011) *The Evidence Base Of Systemic Family and Couples Therapy.* Association of Family Therapy.

Summer J (2015) Live supervision and the 'team without the screen': A home-based approach to training social workers in systemic practice. *Context* **139** 22–27.

Thoburn J (2015) The 'Family Recovery' approach to helping struggling families. In: K Davies (Ed) *Social Work with Troubled Families: A critical introduction* (pp74–99). London: Jessica Kingsley.

Treacher A & Carpenter J (1984) *Using Family Therapy: A guide for practitioners in different professional systems.* Oxford: Basil Blackwell.

Vetere A & Cooper J (2001). Working systemically with family violence: risk, responsibility and collaboration. *Journal of Family Therapy* **23** (4) 378–396.

Walrond-Skinner S (1976) *Family Therapy: The treatment of natural systems.* London: Routledge & Kegan Paul.

Williams L & Auburn T (2015) Accessible polyvocality and paired talk: how family therapists talk positive connotation into being. *Journal of Family Therapy* doi: 10.1111/1467-6427.12096.

Chapter 21

Keeping the family in mind: working together in Liverpool to implement a programme of innovation and change

By Louise Wardale, on behalf of Barnardo's, Liverpool City Council, Liverpool Clinical Commissioning Group, Mersey Care NHS Trust & Liverpool Mental Health Consortium

Introduction

Liverpool is a vibrant, diverse city with many claims to fame – we have two cathedrals, two premier football teams, two Liver Birds and the birthplace of a boy band you may have heard of called the Beatles, to name a few. We are a global city, one that's proud of its heritage and culture, but we are also passionate about looking to the future. We are known for our sense of humour, talking 'scouse' and rallying round to support one another in times of need – and we have experienced many of those.

There is, however, no hiding from the fact that we do experience significant challenges, Liverpool remains the most disadvantaged local authority in England, with just over a third of our children living in poverty, rising to 60% in some areas of the city (Liverpool City Council, 2013a). We know that the rates of common and severe mental ill health are higher in Liverpool than in most other parts of the country (NHS Liverpool CCG, 2014) and that the level of unpaid care provided by children and young people is significantly higher than both regional and national levels (Liverpool City Council, 2013b; Liverpool City Council, 2015d).

As the Mayor of Liverpool stated in the *Liverpool Health and Wellbeing strategy 2014-2019* (Liverpool City Council, 2014), *'Good health and wellbeing is therefore in everyone's interest and indeed, is everyone's responsibility and requires everyone to play their part'*.

We would like to take this opportunity to share the journey we have been on, the part we have been playing, the challenges and the achievements along the way and what works well here in Liverpool in the field of parental mental health and child welfare and beyond.

The 'Think Family' approach and 'Keeping the Family in Mind'

Throughout this chapter you'll read about how the 'Think Family' approach has and continues to be threaded throughout our work, with three essential strands being central to the developments:

1. The importance of relationships.
2. Partnerships.
3. Active participation of children, young people, parents and families.

In Liverpool collectively we have been 'thinking family' for some years and adopting a 'whole family' approach to bring about better outcomes for families here in the city (Liverpool City Council, 2015a; Mersey Care NHS Trust, 2015).

Back in 2001 we launched a small commissioned development project called 'Keeping the Family in Mind' (KFIM) in response to research based in our Liverpool Barnardo's Action with Young Carers Service (Gopfert *et al*, 1999). The project, being located in the Barnado's service, has been a critical success factor as children and young people who are caring for parents with mental health problems are best placed to tell us what works for them and their families. This has been the backbone of the development work from its inception. The service had a track record of involving children and young people who were young carers in decision-making processes and was developing practices to support the whole family by working closely with children and adult services. Put simply, it just made sense (Jackson, 2008).

The research made us take stock of what was really happening and the impact of parental mental health on the whole family. What struck us so powerfully were the concerns of parents experiencing mental distress about the impact on their children's emotional and educational development, their struggle to maintain an adequate parenting role while ill, their grief at being separated from their children if they were admitted to hospital and the lack of support and acknowledgement from adult mental health services that they even had children. The children talked of being ignored by the professionals, of not being informed, of struggling to make sense of their parents' behaviour and of wanting a 'normal' life like that of their peers.

At the time it felt like this was a new way of working, exciting and a great opportunity, but conversely overwhelming, daunting, and it raised questions such as 'can we really bring about improvements, and most importantly, sustainability?' We recognised that without changes in culture and practice within our local health and social care organisations there would be little improvement to provision for children and families who are impacted by mental distress.

Our hypothesis was that a strategic combination of actions was needed, but that the cornerstone of all change must be the participation of children, parents and families.

Bear in mind this was 2001 – it was all uncharted territory and well before the much needed shift in policy that kick started the 'Think Family' approach.

We very much welcomed the *Mental Health and Social Exclusion report* (ODPM, 2004) and in particular what became known as the 'Action 16' of the plan. This focused on enhancing opportunities and outcomes for parents, and their children, with mental health needs (Fowler *et al*, 2009).

Why was change necessary for Liverpool?

We knew the issues around parental mental health and child welfare were shared locally, nationally and internationally, but we needed to really address them if we were really going to make a difference in the city. Sadly we knew that far too often, for families with children and young people under 18, mental health problems represented a significant crisis, not just in terms of parent's individual mental health but family life overall. In our young carers we saw this first hand – parents being hospitalised, everyday routines disrupted and family members overwhelmed and overstretched. Central to this was both parents and children feeing worried and powerless. The evidence at the time was that more than a third of adult service users were parents with dependent children, and the lived experiences illustrated poignantly that some children not only experienced hardship, but even serious risk and fatal harm.

For us it was clear that these families were often caught at the interfaces between service areas and included some of the most disadvantaged and socially excluded people in our communities. Change was needed so that parents could feel less isolated and worried about the effect their illness may have on their children, while children needed to feel less guilty, anxious and over-burdened. Therefore services needed to promote recovery and take into account the effects on the whole family.

So the golden thread was now visible and our senior managers across Liverpool City Council Children's and Adult Services, our local mental health trust (Mersey Care NHS Trust, Child Adolescent Mental Health Services), Alder Hey Children's NHS Foundation Trust, the PCT (as it was then), Liverpool Mental Health Consortium and our Barnardo's 'Keeping Family In Mind' (KFIM) project recognised what has very much remained our core principle: 'Thinking Family' and meeting the needs of families effectively does not lie within the power of a single organisation or service.

This has been very much our mantra to date – it has given us the real impetus as agencies to work together to overturn barriers and improve the responses we can make to parents and their children. No small challenge we'd set ourselves. The gauntlet we threw down was that what we described as one of those categories of work in the 'too hard basket' would be challenged head on and improvements sought and sustained.

How did Liverpool take this forward?

We feel confident in saying that the developments have not happened by accident or in isolation, neither have they been purely process driven. They have grown organically in response to children's, young people's and families' lived experiences; the golden thread was now being given opportunities to weave widely across the systems.

In the early 2000s, the KFIM project was well respected and gathered momentum. However, it was set up as a small development project which contributed to the improvements made in services such as health, education, social care and voluntary organisations when working with children and parents. They live their lives and what we have been advocating continually is that services should have 'open doors' to positively support families along their journeys to ensure better outcomes.

The trick was that KFIM didn't remain a small project in isolation, on the peripheral of issues. Instead, it's best understood as a dynamic and collaborative approach which has been expanded by committed individuals and organisations working together and being flexible about other people coming on board to bring about service and system improvement.

Aim, change outcomes and values: FAMILY

In 2007 with momentum gathering, high levels of energy and key senior support across the city, we set up Families Affected by Mental Ill-health in Liverpool (FAMILY), a collaborative to support implementing the recommendations emerging from a practice survey (led by Care Services Improvement Partnership, Barnardo's Action with Young Carers and KFIM (Barnardo's, CSIP & Pearl Consultancy Services, 2008)). This was a great opportunity to pilot a whole-systems outcomes collaborative and we wanted to reach further into parts of the whole system at multiple levels. It is fair to say that our hypothesis, that this would only have a level of success if we were working collaboratively, was borne out strategically and operationally.

Aim

→ To ensure the continuing development of family-focused polices, services and systems for children and families affected by mental ill health in Liverpool.

Change outcomes

→ Integrated working polices to be developed and implemented to make sure that family's needs and potential were put at the centre.

→ Integrated working practices to be developed and implemented across child and adult systems.

→ Children and families to be supported to fulfil their potential, achieve and maintain health and well-being.

Working values

→ **Service user and carer involvement**
The FAMILY collaborative will seek to ensure the contribution and expertise of parents, carers, children and young people is valued and used in all aspects and at all levels of activity.

→ **Efficiency and sustainability**
To add value to existing review and activity, the FAMILY collaborative will aim to work without duplication or competition.

→ **Interagency working**
Meeting the needs of affected families requires the combined efforts of a wide range of agencies and organisations and the FAMILY collaborative will work jointly with representatives from key sectors and organisations as needed.

→ **Accessibility and discrimination**
The collaborative will be proactive in facilitating the involvement of minority and marginalised groups.

Our methodology and learning

We followed a quality improvement methodology that used Plan, Do, Study, Act (PDSA) cycles in order to test ideas in small increments before change was rolled out into the whole system. We ran a series of learning events with participants from children's services (education, health and social care), Mersey Care NHS Trust (specialist adult mental health), voluntary sector providers, primary care, public health, commissioning and adult social care. Over 200 staff were involved in over 30 PDSA cycles and they produced a rich source of data, providing detailed insights into the efforts and experiences of staff engaging with the challenging task of improvement. One staff member said: *'I found the PDSA cycles helpful in identifying priority areas of work, helped me work through in small chunks that were manageable.'*

The learning events themselves were just as important, characterised by noise and discussion, exchange of ideas and networking:

'As a senior manager, my involvement has been to support the staff working within the FAMILY collaborative and then to observe the opportunities and progress made using the PDSA cycles. This has been a fantastic project to be involved in, reminding us all that worthwhile change doesn't always cost money!'

The whole FAMILY project/approach was documented and it was recognised that the most important point was that service responses in Liverpool to parents (and their children) with mental health difficulties did seem to be improving. We felt confident making this statement as the 'Keeping the Family in Mind' collaborative, by which we meant the combination of the project, its partners and use of innovative improvement methodologies, was characterised by high levels of partnership, ownership, energy and drive.

When the project began, the support from commissioners and senior managers was visible throughout the local authority, the PCT (now Liverpool Clinical Commissioning Group) and the Trusts. We knew then that senior leadership was an important marker of success, particularly when present across systems and focused towards a common goal. We can say with confidence that this has remained critical. Despite internal and external pressures and changes, this support at senior leadership level has been sustained and has played a vital role in our journey. This has resulted in working to tackle issues that were often placed in the 'too hard basket' with lids firmly shut.

We often use the word 'partnership' casually, as if it is a phenomenon that just somehow happens. However we have learnt first-hand that the vital ingredients for effective partnership working include time, commitment, trust and patience, to name a few. Acknowledging the 'elephant in the room' and being honest, we have asked ourselves 'What's in it for me and my organisation, how will this help me in my role and the families I work with, is this going to take me away from my core duties?'

What was becoming so evident at the time from the FAMILY collaborative learning and all the KFIM work was that partnerships are crucial to success: 'different agenda, shared goal'. Central to this is the partnership with services and service users and carers – particularly children, young people, young carers and their parents – and was summed up very succinctly at the collaborative as: *'Families' experiences show us what needs to be changed in conversations with practitioners and managers – working it out together'* (Barnados, CSIP & Pearl Consultancy Services, 2008).

Outcomes and improvements

We know that there is still much to do and that improvements are continuous. Earlier we highlighted Action 16 of the Mental Health and Social Exclusion Plan (ODPM, 2014), which focused on 'improving opportunities and outcomes for parents with mental health needs and their children'. This review was produced in 2009, but is worth mentioning as much of our work was highlighted and this allowed us to take stock of the achievements up to that point. Much of what we outline below has since been built on further, continually bedded in and responding to local needs and changes.

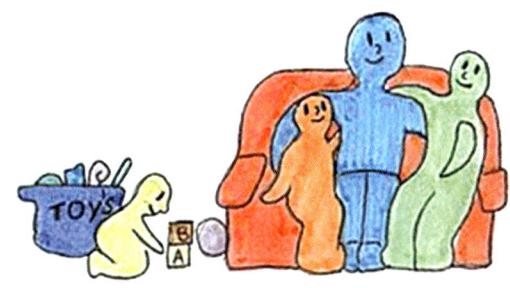

Jelly baby logo

This is our Kite-Mark illustrating that the standard is met for family-orientated services e.g. family rooms and child-friendly literature. It was designed by young carers supported by Barnardo's KFIM and is a brand in its own right. This is the official seal of approval that the young carers award and testimony that they are at the heart of improvements.

Culture changes

It is always hard to claim how this can be measured – though we feel that we have had some successes, which include the above Kite Mark, and the fact that family rooms are part and parcel of all Mersey Care inpatient provision is testimony to this. There are 16 family rooms in total, from the local services through to low, medium and high secure services. We are proud of how we worked together and developed the first family room back in 2001 and how this has been a response to delivering services that really do place families at the heart; their experiences have rightly been given centre stage. We do consistently evaluate and improve the family room provision, never sitting back in the ignorant belief that the work is done, and quotes such as this illustrate their importance:

> 'You need your mum, and when she has to go to hospital she does not stop being your mum, and you are still a kid, no matter how grown up you think you are… Your head is full of all sorts, but somehow just having that room and decent staff just sort of helps you feel people do care and do understand. I am so pleased that our views got listened to and we can help other families too… thank you!'
> (Robinson & Scott, 2007; ADASS & ADCS, 2011; Mersey Care NHS Trust, 2011)

Increased visibility, improved identification

In 2007 we undertook a local and national anti-stigma postcard campaign. The series of postcards all had powerful messages from young carers and children impacted by parental mental ill health (Wardale, 2007).

Our 'Message in a Bottle' scheme was initially piloted in a Mersey Care community mental health team and then rolled out. With permission from the Lions Trust, we personalised their bottles and made them more child-friendly. We developed this emergency planning tool to support children and parents to plan together in advance of crisis situations so their needs can be best meet in line with their wishes and requests, so they are at the centre of the planning. We recently updated this with young carers and parents leading the way to make sure it works best for them.

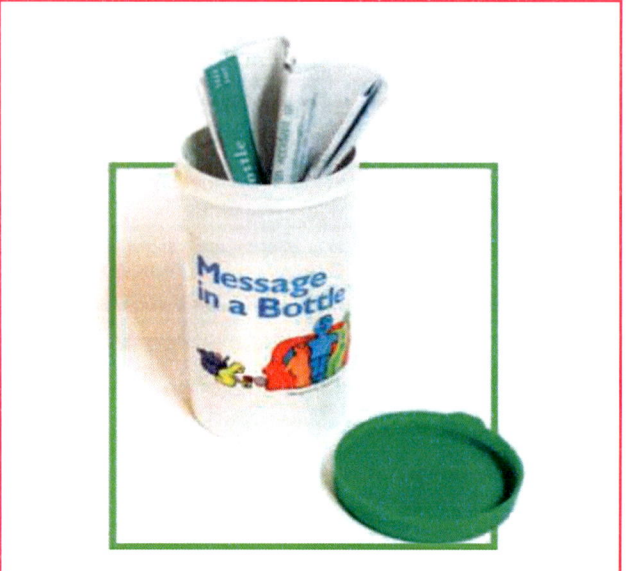

Improving access to support and services

This has included the implementation of Mersey Care procedures such as the notification letter for parents with children under five that is sent from the care co-ordinator to the health visitor. This has now been extended to a letter to the school health practitioner for children over five-years old.

Improved access to assessments

A number of years ago we developed a young carers assessment and care planning policy and procedure which stated that adult workers should undertake the young carers assessment as part of support to the adult. The policy and guidance was developed by the Liverpool City Council in partnership with Barnardo's Liverpool, Mersey Care NHS Trust, Sefton MBC and Sefton Young Carers Project and, as such, is a joint policy with Mersey Care NHS Trust, who undertakes Young Carers Assessments on behalf of Liverpool City Council. The council and its partners are now reviewing their young carers' assessment policy and guidance in line with both the Care Act (2014) and the Children and Families Act (2014). Although in the early stages, the pathway will be embedded within our Early Help Assessment Framework.

Taking our learning forward

There is little doubt that Liverpool's collaborative way of working and strong senior commitment led to the city's involvement with Social Care Institute for Excellence's (SCIE) guide *Think Child, Think Parent, Think Family: A guide to parental mental health and child welfare* (SCIE, 2009). In 2009, Liverpool was chosen by SCIE to be an implementation site for what simply became known as the 'Think Family' guide. We were one of five sites nationally selected on the basis of promising practice. This was very much welcomed and allowed us to further raise awareness and continue to give priority to the agenda of delivering high-quality services for families by taking a multi-agency approach and working across both child and adult services to achieve better outcomes for families. This has allowed us to continue exploring ways of working with the whole family when parents are identified as having mental ill health.

Our 'Think Family' implementation work is promoted on the SCIE website (http://www.scie.org.uk/children/parentalmentalhealthandchildwelfare/implementation.asp) (SCIE, 2015).

We were able to shine a light on the gaps and push forward on service improvement in the areas we had described as 'too hard'. Of significance has been the development of Mersey Care Family Support Workers (FSW) in community mental health teams. This initiative, which we have evaluated and continue to monitor and improve, is testimony to strategic partnership working, including our children centres, CAMHS – Alder Hey, CCG Commissioning, Barnardo's and Liverpool City Council. The FSWs work directly with parents and their children who are supported by Mersey Care, working to a whole family approach and utilising the Family Outcome Star.

Early Help

Our Early Help offer and turning around the lives of families with multiple and complex needs in the city have been influenced and informed by our earlier learning and the energy we have dedicated to parental mental health and child welfare. Our KFIM collaborative and SCIE implementation have allowed us to explore, test and improve, which has certainly helped to engage partners, share ownership and support closer joint working across adults and children systems.

We have made sure that there is strong alignment and 'read across' all our strategies, policies and procedures with children's, parents and family's needs viewed in the wider framework of the 'Think Child, Think Parent, Think Family, Think Community' model.

From 2010 until now, we have continued to learn and develop our Liverpool 'Think Family' approach and what we now more commonly describe as a 'Whole Family' approach. This is to support the family, taking into account the individual needs and the combined needs of the child, parent and other family members. The strong evidence base demonstrated throughout this chapter firmly supports what we know quite simply to be a sensible and extremely effective approach for us here in the city.

During this time as a Liverpool partnership we were awarded Department of Education funding for 18 months under the Carers Trust Integrated Intervention Programme, along with seven other partnerships around England. The overall aim of the programme was for *'partnership sites to adopt an inclusive and whole family approach that prevents or reduces the amount of excessive or harmful caring undertaken by young carers under 18 in England' (Fletcher, 2015)*. We were able to build further on our implementation of the SCIE guide and improve multi-agency approaches to better identify and support young carers and their families, where there was parental illness or disability.

We continued to partner with services across health, social care, education, public health and the voluntary sector to more effectively identify, integrate and support young carers and their families. This included developing our Adult's and Children's Family Assessment and Pathway, building on Team Around the Family approaches and working with strategic partners in the city. Working together, we promoted and embedded the *Memorandum Of Understanding for Young Carers* (MOU) (ADASS & ADCS, 2009) across adult and children's services with the aim of *'making this a reality between the partner organisations'* (ADASS & ADCS, 2009). It was evident that the strategic focus of the partnership was heavily guided by the KFIM work that we, as partners, had been jointly working on. KFIM's role was valued as being that of a 'critical friend' and being the glue that binds.

This was reinforced as the work was independently evaluated and the report (Peter Fletcher Associates) outlined how Liverpool had increased the opportunities for effective communication, had strong ownership and involvement of key decision makers and senior managers (Fletcher, 2015). It was also recognised that our strategic impact was a result of us aligning the work with existing and new policy agendas and finding the fit.

This was critical during this timeframe, as the Liverpool Families programme (Liverpool City Council, 2015c) began in April 2013, and the work has been able to further develop as a result of the learning to date. This strategic work programme across Liverpool City Council and partner agencies has allowed us to embed a family focus in the design, delivery and development of services to families in Liverpool in order to improve outcomes and reduce costs. The ambition is for families in Liverpool to have resourcefulness and resilience along with the attitude, skills and behaviours that will enable them and the city to thrive.

We are currently implementing our Early Help strategy (Liverpool City Council, 2015b) and we know from experience that this is about changing culture and all of our partners making a commitment to work differently, which takes time. We have learnt by listening and working with families that adopting a whole systems approach to service redesign is critical if we are to make sure families receive early help as soon as difficulties emerge. We want to respond as soon as possible when difficulties emerge so we can prevent problems from becoming entrenched or escalating.

Much work has focused on developing our revised Early Help Assessment arrangements. This has led us to a move away from the Common Assessment Framework to the Family Early Help Assessment Tool and we are now developing three locality-based Early Help Hubs.

Workforce development

Multi-agency workforce development and culture change have remained central throughout the journey. We aim to share a consistent message about what is needed to support a 'Whole Family' approach when working in multi-agency settings. This means educating the workforce about the benefits of working to a 'Whole Family' approach when working with families or commissioning services, and to have the skills, confidence and knowledge to effectively challenge and support families and partners. To date, over 1,700 practitioners have been trained up as Early Help Assessment Tool (EHAT) lead professionals and a 'train the trainer' programme is being developed so that agencies and services can take ownership and lead the multi-agency sessions as a sustainable way forward. Many of the developments have been spring boarded from our SCIE Think Family and Integrated Interventions learning, in particular how adult services, including mental health services (along with GPs, police and fire and rescue services), are now using pre-EHATs to prompt a multi-agency response to need and helping families navigate through the system, ensuring early help support is offered. This is a timely reminder that our mantra of *'Thinking Family and meeting the needs of families effectively does not lie within the gift of a single organisation or service'* is more critical now than ever.

Hopefully this gives you a flavour of how we have been working together across the city. We are not complacent, and though our strategic approach and direction along with policies and procedures may all be aligned, we fully recognise that we need to continually assess, review and evaluate working practices.

The 'golden thread' of 'Thinking Family' has continued to weave in and out, tying together what we do and how we do it to ensure strong connectivity and prevent gaps widening. Those essential strands of partnership, relationships and the effectiveness and importance of listening to families (particularly children and young people) cannot be overstated. We fully recognise that whole family working is both a challenge and an imperative, and we remain steadfast and committed to build on its developments to date. We know that collaboration and ensuring that any changes which happen are informed by the voices and experiences of children, young people and their families is vital. And we also know that relatively small changes can make huge differences to families' experiences.

Our final words go to Chloe, aged 16 years old…

> 'Being a young carer is not down to choice – it just happens – it is what it is – asking for help isn't easy but what helps is when services for adults and children work together. I can tell you first hand that there is no magic wand but for me and my family, we were not asking for big things – getting the support for us took time from the professionals and trust on our side – but when it works well and it can, then it makes all the difference for all my family.'

References

ADASS & ADCS (2009) *Working Together to Support Young Carers: A model local memorandum of understanding between statutory directors for children's services and adult social services* [online]. London: Association of Directors of Adult Services & Association of Directors of Children's Services. Available at: http://www.adass.org.uk/adassmedia/stories/MOU%20Working%20Together%20to%20support%20young%20carers.pdf (accessed November 2015).

ADASS & ADCS (2011) *Signposts: See me, hear me, talk to me – talk to my family as well* [online]. Association of Directors of Children's Services. Available at: http://lx.iriss.org.uk/content/signposts-see-me-hear-me-talk-me-talk-my-family-well (accessed November 2015).

Barnardo's, CSIP and Pearl Consultancy Services (2008) *Liverpool FAMILY Collaborative: Update on Activity*.

Fletcher P (2015) *Final Report: Evaluation of the Integrated Interventions Programme for Carers Trust* [online]. London: Carers Trust. Available at: https://makingastepchangepractice.files.wordpress.com/2015/06/final-report-evaluation-of-the-integrated-interventions-programme-for-carers-trust.pdf (accessed November 2015).

Fowler R, Robinson B & Scott S (2009) *Improving Opportunities and Outcomes for Parents with Mental Health Needs and Their Children* [online]. Available at: http://www.barnardos.org.uk/action16-2.pdf (accessed November 2015).

Gopfert M, Harrison P & Mahoney C (1999) *Keeping the Family in Mind: Participative research into mental ill-health & how it affects the whole family*. Liverpool: North Mersey Community NHS Trust.

Jackson C (2008) 'Me when I cheer my mummy up by dancing'. *Mental Health Today* (May 2008, p.16-18).

Liverpool City Council (2013a) *Children and Young Peoples Plan 2013-2017* [online]. Available at: http://liverpool.gov.uk/media/80533/children-and-young-peoples-plan.pdf (accessed November 2015).

Liverpool City Council (2013b) *Population Groups: Young carers* [online]. Available at: http://liverpool.gov.uk/media/688873/populationgroupscarersyoungpeople.pdf (accessed November 2015).

Liverpool City Council (2014) *Liverpool Health and Wellbeing Strategy 2014-2019*. Liverpool City Council.

Liverpool City Council (2015a) *Think Family* [online]. Available at: http://liverpool.gov.uk/council/strategies-plans-and-policies/children-and-families/think-family/ (accessed November 2015).

Liverpool City Council (2015b) *Early Help Strategy* [online]. Available at: http://liverpool.gov.uk/council/strategies-plans-and-policies/children-and-families/early-help-strategy/ (accessed November 2015).

Liverpool City Council (2015c) *Liverpool Families Programme* [online]. Available at: http://liverpool.gov.uk/council/strategies-plans-and-policies/children-and-families/liverpool-families-programme/ (accessed November 2015).

Liverpool City Council (2015d) *Joint Strategic Needs Assessment* [online]. Available at: http://liverpool.gov.uk/council/strategies-plans-and-policies/adult-services-and-health/joint-strategic-needs-assessment/ (accessed November 2015).

Mersey Care NHS Trust (2011) *Family Rooms Review 2012* [online]. Available at: http://www.merseycare.nhs.uk/media/1066/family-rooms-review-2012.pdf (accessed November 2015).

Mersey Care NHS Trust (2014) *Think Family: Progress report* [online]. Available at: http://www.merseycare.nhs.uk/our-services/think-family/ (accessed November 2015).

Mersey Care NHS Trust (2015) *Supporting Your Whole Family* [online]. Available at: http://www.merseycare.nhs.uk/our-services/think-family/ (accessed November 2015).

NHS Liverpool CCG (2014) *Liverpool Primary Mental Health Care Strategy for Adults: 2013-2016* [online]. Available at: http://www.liverpoolccg.nhs.uk/Library/Health_and_Services/Mental_Health/Liverpool%20Primary%20Mental%20Health%20Care%20Strategy%20for%20Adults%202013%20to%202016.pdf (accessed November 2015).

Office of the Deputy Prime Minister (2004) *Mental Health and Social Exclusion Report* [online]. London. HMSO. Available at: http://www.nfao.org/Useful_Websites/MH_Social_Exclusion_report_summary.pdf (accessed November 2015).

Robinson B & Scott S (2007) *Parents in Hospital: How mental health services can best promote family contact when a parent is in hospital* [online]. Barnardos. Available at: http://www.barnardos.org.uk/resources/research_and_publications/parents-in-hospital-how-mental-health-services-can-best-promote-family-contact-when-a-parent-is-in-hospital/publication-view.jsp?pid=PUB-1393 (accessed 2015).

SCIE (2009) *Think Child, Think Parent, Think Family: A guide to parental mental health and child welfare* [online]. Available at: http://www.scie.org.uk/publications/guides/guide30/ (accessed August 2015).

SCIE (2015) *Parental Mental Health and Child Welfare* [online]. Available at: http://www.scie.org.uk/children/parentalmentalhealthandchildwelfare/resources.asp (accessed November 2015).

Wardale L (2007) *Keeping the Family in Mind – resource pack*. Liverpool: Barnados. Available for purchase at: http://www.barnardos.org.uk/resources/research_and_publications/keeping-the-family-in-mind-resource-pack-2nd-edition/publication-view.jsp?pid=PUB-1600 (accessed November 2015).

Chapter 22
Think Family, Northern Ireland
By Mary Donaghy

Introduction

In families where a parent has mental health issues, the mental health and well-being of children and other adults are closely linked to these issues. Not all such families need health and social care services, but those that do often struggle to get accessible and effective support that addresses children's needs and recognises the parental responsibilities of many adults with mental health issues (SCIE, 2012).

In Northern Ireland there have been a number of cases where children have been seriously injured or have died. Enquiries into the circumstances surrounding these cases identified contributing factors to be a combination of parental mental health issues, and deficits in communication and joint working between professionals and agencies. This suggested that the way in which these services work together needed to be improved.

The Department of Health, Social Services and Public Safety (DHSSPS) in Northern Ireland funded two project managers for three years to lead the implementation of a plan to address these issues. Between April 2009 and March 2012 the Mental Health and Children's Services 'Think Child, Think Parent, Think Family' Project worked with adult, mental health and children's services in the statutory and voluntary sectors across Northern Ireland. The project vision was to improve outcomes for parents with mental health issues and their children by establishing a Think Child, Think Parent, Think Family approach to the planning and delivery of services.

Focus

The Think Family project focused on improving collaborative working and enhancing understanding of multi-disciplinary roles and responsibilities of all stakeholders working across the mental health and children's services interface. Introducing the Family Model (Falkov, 1998) as a beneficial conceptual tool has assisted staff in thinking about different family members, their relationships with each other and the impact of external environmental factors. A key concept of the project was to harness and strengthen what is already happening with a Think Family approach.

In July 2009, the Northern Ireland project joined, as a regional pilot site, a national initiative led by the Social Care Institute for Excellence (SCIE) aimed at making improvements in the provision of services when working with parents with mental illness and their children. SCIE published guidance (SCIE, 2011) to assist staff working with parents with mental health problems and their children. The guidance identified what needed to change, making recommendations to improve service planning and delivery, and ultimately to improve outcomes for families. The guidance, which was initially published in 2009 and then revised and updated in 2011, provided a framework for implementation of this important initiative within Northern Ireland.

Recommendations

There are nine priority recommendations identified within *Think Child, Think Parent, Think Family: A guide to parental mental health and child welfare* (SCIE, 2011). These recommendations draw together the best of current practice alongside a renewed emphasis on thinking about families. The recommendations are:

- → signposting and improving access to services
- → screening
- → assessment
- → planning care
- → providing care
- → reviewing care plans
- → strategic approach
- → workforce development
- → gathering more evidence about what works.

The implementation of the project has, to an extent, followed a linear process using these nine recommendations as its framework. Plans were agreed with specific outcomes, which were then implemented and progress reviewed. The process has also been organic in nature, responding to opportunities and changes in the practice and policy environment. Changing attitudes and ways of working takes time, and future progress will require continued commitment from organisations, managers and practitioners/clinicians.

Throughout the Think Family Project, substantial progress was made in seizing every opportunity to embed a Think Family approach into new and existing regional and local initiatives, policies, guidance, training and structures. However, there is still a need to further change organisational culture and understanding of what falls within individuals' remits, supported by senior management to ensure the necessary changes continue.

Structure (2009–2012)

The Think Family project structure consisted of a project board comprised of senior management from relevant adult and children's statutory and voluntary organisations, and service users and carers. Project board members provided overall direction and guidance and were responsible for developing and embedding the Think Family approach in their own organisations. They also attended a workshop to prepare them for their role. The workshop focused on testing their values and ensuring commitment to the task at hand.

Project Locality Teams (PLTs) were established across the five health and social care trust areas which were representative of statutory and voluntary organisations, and service users and carers. In order to do this, two regional workshops were delivered to create initial awareness and discussion on how to move forward. Regular meetings were also held with the five chairs of the PLTs to maintain motivation, focus action plans and address challenges along the way.

Each PLT developed an action plan for their locality based on the first six SCIE recommendations, while the two project managers specifically focused upon recommendations seven and eight. Recommendation nine, gathering more evidence about what works, will be part of phase two of Think Family, where evaluation is a specific work area within the regional action plan. This work will be supported by Dr Adrian Falkov and others (phase two is discussed further later).

PLT chairs were ultimately responsible for driving forward planning and delivery of the changes required to implement the SCIE recommendations. This structure facilitated a consistent approach to change and promoted learning across the project locality team.

A range of activities were undertaken at a regional and local level to implement the SCIE recommendations. These activities are summarised below under each priority recommendation.

Recommendation one: signposting and access to services

In implementing the first recommendation, the PLTs considered how best to provide information for service users, their children and family members, and the general public, in a positive way without further stigmatisation of this client group. The focus was on promoting a positive message about accessing support, reviewing staff perceptions as a mechanism to change attitudes, and developing staff awareness of the full spectrum of services available relating to mental health, parental support and support for children.

Outcomes
- Development of a communication strategy, clearly setting out the aims and objectives of the project.
- Organisation of a publicity campaign, linked with other information activities across the region, to promote a positive message about accessing support as a means of addressing the stereotypes, stigma and fears that the public may have about accessing mental health and children's services.
- Publication of Think Family project newsletters to raise awareness of the project. These were distributed among all staff in services related to mental health and children throughout Northern Ireland to improve their knowledge of the full spectrum of services available relating to mental health, parental support and support for children.
- Development of the Health and Social Care Board's (HSCB) Think Family Project webpage, which provided information relating to the project such as local contacts, local events and changes to service delivery, newsletters and support information for service users and staff: http://www.hscboard.hscni.net/Thinkfamily/.

Involving service users

Meaningful engagement with service users and staff who provide the services was essential to the success of the project. This was achieved by developing a regional voluntary organisation subgroup that supported and provided services to service users and carers.

A specific piece of work completed with this group was the Family and Staff Experience Sense Maker surveys. Parents with mental health issues, their children, carers and staff were asked to complete a survey. They detailed their experiences of services and measured their experience against predefined signifiers using a question framework. Ninety-eight family experiences and 280 staff surveys were completed and the findings are listed below:

- Communication and information sharing between families and professionals, although improved, still remained a concern for many respondents.
- Professional commitment to patient confidentiality overriding the information needs of the family was cited as a reason for poor communication, leading to little or no consultation with family members and questions being left unanswered.
- Children indicated that not being informed or included in the planning process caused anxiety, fear and feelings of isolation. Service users, their children and carers clearly indicated that not understanding the parent's condition negatively impacted on families, especially children.
- Results from the survey indicated that where the needs of the ill parent and children/family members were considered jointly by staff involved, it led to better recovery for the parent, positive outcomes for both parent and children, and greater levels of service satisfaction.

Results of the surveys have influenced and directed ongoing developments within Phase two of the Think Family work in Northern Ireland.

Recommendation two: screening

A major aim of the project was to ensure that the Think Family model was embedded into practice through systems that routinely and reliably identified and recorded information about adults with mental health issues who are parents, as well as their children and family members. This ensured that, from the outset of engagement with the family, screening processes elicited the right information for appropriate assessments and referrals or supports to be offered to meet the families' needs.

Outcomes
- Revision of existing screening/assessment tools across maternity, mental health and children's services to promote a family model approach to the assessment and treatment process at a local and regional level.
- Development and circulation of a list of age-appropriate resources to assist staff and parents in talking to children about mental illness.

Recommendations three to six: assessment and planning, providing and reviewing care

Through a series of workshops, using the SCIE priority recommendations relating to assessment and planning, providing and reviewing care, staff identified the changes required to improve service provision, with each PLT area developing an action plan to address the identified changes.

To guide and support staff to more effective partnership working, a regional adult and children's joint protocol was developed (HSCB, 2011). The protocol set out the principles and best practice guidelines that staff must consider when responding to the needs of parents with mental health issues, including substance misuse, and their children and families. This is set in the context of promoting a Family Model through a collaborative approach to service delivery and effective communication between all stakeholders. The protocol promotes that families affected by mental health issues may benefit from the provision of support and intervention at an earlier stage, thus preventing children becoming 'at risk', and enhancing recovery.

Understanding the Needs of Children in Northern Ireland

Understanding the Needs of Children in Northern Ireland (UNOCINI) is a regional comprehensive assessment process and is also used as the basis for referrals to statutory children's services to identify the needs of children. A review of the UNOCINI guidance for staff highlighted that parental mental health was not explicitly covered. The guidance did not provide for the detailed elements of parental mental health that staff needed to consider when completing an assessment of a parent who has mental health issues.

UNOCINI was revised and an appendix developed to better reflect what practitioners should know and take recognition of when completing an UNOCINI assessment when a parent has mental ill health issues.

Outcomes

→ Development of a Regional Joint Protocol to facilitate joint working between adult mental health and children's services.

→ Development of UNOCINI appendix 1, *A Guide to Understanding the Effect of Parental Mental Health on Children and the Family* (2011)

Recommendation seven: strategic approach

At a strategic level there was a contribution to a number of ongoing initiatives aimed at ensuring the Think Family approach principles were consistently incorporated into the development and planning of services. Key regional initiatives are listed below:

→ Bamford Task Group.

→ Hidden Harm Quality Assurance Group.

→ Children and Young Peoples Strategic partnership.

→ Promoting Quality Care Implementation Groups.

→ Card Before You Leave.

→ Mental Health Service Framework.

→ Children's Services Framework.

→ Perinatal Mental Health Implementation Strategy.

→ Area Child Protection Committee training sub group.

Recommendation eight: workforce development

As health and social care services, systems and practices develop it is important that training and workforce development are in place to provide staff with the necessary knowledge and skills to embed a Think Family approach into practice.

Outcomes

A range of workforce development activities ran during the project. These included:

→ Awareness raising.

→ Inclusion of the Think Family approach into existing training.

→ Practitioner champions groups were established across three of the health and social care trusts.

→ Development of SCIE e-learning materials.

→ A customised multidisciplinary training course for managers focusing on the skills needed to implement a Think Family approach. Risk management processes have to be developed to be provided regionally.

→ Development of a knowledge and skills framework.

→ Liaison with higher education institutions to incorporate the Think Family principles into existing professional training programmes.

Outcome/performance measures

With support from the Health and Social Care Board (HSCB), indicators were developed. These were based on primary data collected from service user and staff family experience surveys and case file audits. Ten services from each of the five trusts were asked to complete a self-audit of case notes set against SCIE good practice standards:

→ Gateway services.

→ Family intervention service.

→ Public health nursing (health visiting).

→ School nursing.

→ Child and adolescent mental health service.

→ Maternity services.

→ Community mental health services.

→ Acute inpatient mental health services.

→ Addiction services.

→ Forensic services.

The returns received numbered 215 with approximately 25 returns per service regionally. Although this was a relatively small audit, results were consistent across services and trusts. From the audit, evidence clearly showed that services were beginning to assess the impact of mental illness on the wider family.

Results also indicated that staff were beginning to consider how mental illness can impact upon family life. However, the typical case work model of engagement was between the individual and professionals, with little or no engagement with the wider family system. Within case files/records there was limited evidence to suggest that carers were consistently being communicated with or involved in the planning and delivery of care.

Case files/records showed that children were talked about but not talked to, and weren't included in the care of their parent. Where cases were set within formal child protection procedures the needs of children were considered within the case conference plan. But again there was limited evidence to suggest that children had been given information relating to their parent's mental illness or that the children had been included in the planning and delivery of care for their parent.

Recommendations for future work

Further change to organisational culture and peoples' understanding of what falls within their remit is required. There were also some key barriers that were encountered which would benefit from further investigation:

- → Further exploration to ensure a clear care pathway exists for families where a parent experiences mental ill health. This should include identification and the needs of families who fall into the 'lower level' support.
- → Technical solutions to link up children's services databases with mental health databases to assist in the identification and assessment of need for families and children.
- → Although outcome/performance measures were developed on a smaller scale, more robust measurement of indicators and evaluation is essential.
- → Information sharing is critical at all stages of the care pathway. Trusts/organisations need to consider how staff communicate relevant information/explanations about mental illness and the impact on family life to carers and children, either directly or through their parents/carers in an age-appropriate manner.
- → Future work to ensure Think Family principles are embedded in professional education at all levels.

Think Family NI (2014) – phase two

When the Think Child, Think Parent, Think Family Project ended in October 2012, it became core business for the HSCB. Phase two of the Think Family work is now under the structure of Children & Young Peoples Strategic Partnership (CYPSP) which is led by the HSCB (http://cypsp.org/).

A new dimension brought to the work is the development of Think Family in its widest context that includes not only dependent children and young people of parents with mental health issues, but also those adult carers who continue to care for their adult children who have mental health issues.

A regional workshop was held to develop thinking around how phase two of Think Family should commence. A regional Think Family subgroup was developed consisting of adult mental health, children's and voluntary organisations from existing and new membership. Terms of reference were developed, which clearly focused on learning from the project. The focus of the work has been based on realistic achievements to ensure that the benefits are meaningful for families and that it clearly makes a difference for them.

An exciting development for phase two of Think Family is the achievement of commissioned support from Dr Adrian Falkov, author of *The Family Model Handbook* (Falkov, 2012). The Family Model will be used in Northern Ireland as the framework in a pilot project taking place in the South Eastern Health and Social Care Trust. The pilot project will make the necessary changes using the Family Model to build upon and strengthen a family focus. Dr Falkov has delivered two regional conferences in Northern Ireland and is currently providing support to the pilot project, which is a specific area of work stemming from the regional Think Family Action Plan.

Regional Think Family Action Plan

The Regional Action Plan is based on learning from the family and staff experience surveys undertaken within the Think Child, Think Parent, Think Family Project. The themes from the surveys are:

- → Improved communication between professionals and families.
- → Improved access to early intervention family support for children, young people and their families.
- → Improving the extent to which assessment, planning and treatment are inclusive of a 'whole family' approach.

All of the above will form the basis of our work for the future combined with robust evaluation that will be taken forward in partnership with academics and practitioners.

What have we done to date?

- → Developed leaflets for children and young people giving them information about mental health issues relating to their parents and carers.
- → Launched the children's and young people's leaflets in each health and social care trust area and provided awareness sessions relating to phase two of the Think Family work.
- → Continued to ensure that Think Family shapes and influences strategic direction. This allows a strengthening of collaboration at this level so that partnership approaches to regional changes reflect a Think Family approach.
- → Developed performance indicators using a recognised methodology to measure areas within the regional action plan. This work is being taken forward in partnership with Dr Adrian Falkov, the Safeguarding Board Northern Ireland, academic institutions and practitioners, and will form an important and integral part of Phase 2 Think Family work.
- → The pilot project in the South Eastern Health & Social Care Trust is made up of adult mental health, addiction, acute inpatient, children's and three voluntary organisations and started in September 2014, covering a period of two years and occurring in three stages.

Stage one

Stage one will strengthen documentation in the above service areas with information from Children of Parents with Mental illness (COPMI) (http://www.copmi.net.au/). During the Think Child, Think Parent, Think Family project, information from COPMI was used to strengthen documentation within various service areas. During phase two, COPMI information is being used to strengthen documentation further and the revised Family Model is the continued framework being used to support staff in family focused practice.

How will this work?

- Staff will begin to use the strengthened documentation upon initial referral for all families presenting.
- Those that need lower level family support will be referred to the family support hubs that have been developed under CYPSP. This starts the process of changing the culture of how you think and practise.
- Those families who are assessed as needing further involvement from the community mental health and/or addiction team will continue to get a family focused approach.
- If the person's mental health/addiction issues deteriorate the family focus will continue during their admission into the acute inpatient ward/addiction ward in the Downe sector of South Eastern HSC Trust.
- On discharge from the inpatient ward, the Community Mental Health and/or Addiction Team will continue their involvement and provide a family focused approach using the Family Model concept.

Stage two

Stage two will focus primarily on adult mental health (AMH) staff having the family conversation. This includes increasing the knowledge and skills of AMH staff to make the family focus their core business.

How will this work?

- AMH staff will have specific training to build their knowledge and skills in talking to children and young people.
- Upon referral to AMH services, staff will engage the person in conversation reflecting on questions in the strengthened assessment and review documentation.
- Voluntary partners in the pilot will assist AMH staff to have conversations with children and young people and with adult carers to begin the process of the family conversation.
- This process will allow families to become involved from the outset in assessment, planning and review of their care, building upon the importance of the strengths and support within the family, as appropriate.

Stage three

Stage three will focus on the environment of the facilities, including upgrading family rooms in the addiction and acute inpatient ward to allow family visits to occur in a more stimulating environment that enhances engagement for the parent and their dependants.

How will this work?

- Voluntary organisations will use their existing young carers group to agree how and what should be provided in the family rooms in addictions and inpatient wards.
- Local facilities will be used for family conversations to reduce stigma and enhance motivation.
- Develop a Think Family social assessment for use by social work staff using the Family Model domains.

In conclusion

Phase two of Think Family is an exciting and challenging development for Northern Ireland. We may not achieve all that we hope for, but in doing all of this work the emphasis has to be on including the family in conversation. If the focus on the family continues as a priority, by listening to what families want, need and how they can help in the recovery of their parent or carer, it will make a difference.

Using the Family Model as a framework will give focus and purpose to the development of this work. The commitment and willingness of organisations, management and staff in Northern Ireland to change their thinking and practice to become family focused at every level has already begun. There is more to do and it will be a journey that will see success and challenges, however, if we accomplish what we set out to do we will have achieved and delivered a more meaningful service to families.

For more information on Think Family go to www.cypsp.org

References

Falkov A (1998) *Crossing Bridges: Training resources for working with mentally ill parents and their children – Reader for managers, practitioners and trainers*. Brighton: Pavilion Publishing.

Falkov A (2012) *The Family Model Handbook: An integrated approach to supporting mentally ill parents and their children*. Brighton: Pavilion Publishing.

Health and Social Care Board (HSCB) (2011) Adult and Children's Services Joint Protocol: *Responding to the needs of children whose parents have mental health and/or substance misuse issues*.

SCIE (2011) *Think Child, Think Parent, Think Family: A guide to parental mental health and child welfare (Revised)* [online]. London: SCIE. Available at: http://www.scie.org.uk/publications/guides/guide30/ (accessed October 2015).

SCIE (2012) *Think Child, Think Parent, Think Family: Final evaluation report*. London: SCIE.

UNOCINI (2011) *A Guide to understanding the effect of parental mental health on children and the family* [online]. Available at: http://www.dhsspsni.gov.uk/microsoft_word_-_a_guide_to_understanding_the_effect_of_parental_mh_on_children_and_their_family_june_2011-2.pdf (accessed October 2015).

Research digest

Research digest

Paul David Spencer Ross

Introduction

The abstracts contained within this digest cover recently published research studies from 2012 to 2015 on parental mental health and child welfare. Each study listed in this research digest will include a URL to the full research study or abstract including information on how to search for current evidence on parental mental health and child welfare using a database or search engine.

The research contained within the digest has been selected to highlight both the topics discussed in this annual and examples of research not included, but still relevant to the overall topic. Due to a diverse range of research on parental mental health and child welfare, it has been impossible to include everything, but this digest offers a snapshot of current research and the reader is recommended to conduct their own searches.

This research digest has been compiled using SCIE's Social Care Online, *'the UK's largest database of information and research on all aspects of social care and social work'* (SCIE) and through subject expert recommendations.

To find up-to-date research on parental mental health and child welfare, visit social care online using the following search terms: parental mental health and children, in either the basic or advanced search facility, or you could visit Google Scholar or ProQuest Databases such as PsycINFO, or publisher journal sites such as Pavilion, Wiley, Ingentaconnect, Taylor & Francis or Emerald etc. For additional tips and hints to conduct further searching on the topic, see Ross PDS (2015) for more information.

Research abstracts

1. **Mixed methods study with 69 participants (8-12 year olds) reviewing the impact of peer support programmes, such as telephone helplines, in relation to children's experience of change and discusses its core ingredients.**

Grove C, Reupert A & Maybery D (2015) Peer connections as an intervention with children of families where a parent has a mental illness: moving towards an understanding of the processes of change. *Children and Youth Services Review* 48 177–185.

Prevention and early intervention programmes have been found to impede the transmission of mental illness from parents to children. However, the extant processes of change in such programmes are less clear.

This study focuses on the impact of a peer support programme developed for children and adolescents who have a parent with a mental illness and examines the processes of change that might promote positive outcomes for them.

A mixed methods research approach was employed with participants aged between eight and 12 years old; 69 completed pre- and post-questionnaires and 18 of these same participants engaged in telephone interviews post programme.

Results demonstrate improved mental health knowledge, and children reported that they were more likely to use an anonymous telephone helpline after attending the programme. Children indicated that the programme provided a place of respite from caring for their parent with a mental illness, an opportunity to connect with peers, and a positive change in perception of their parent's mental illness.

The reported findings are moving towards an understanding of the process of change in programmes.

2. **Psychiatric rehabilitation and recovery-based intervention pilot study for parents with severe mental illnesses containing perspectives from both parents and practitioners in relation to outcomes and affects to quality of life.**

van der Ende PC, van Busschbach JT, Nicholson J, Korevaar EL & van Weeghel J (2014) Parenting and psychiatric rehabilitation: can parents with severe mental illness benefit from a new approach? *Psychiatric Rehabilitation Journal* 37 (3) 201–208.

Objective: The aim of this pilot implementation study was to explore the initial experiences with and impact of Parenting with Success and Satisfaction (PARSS), a psychiatric rehabilitation and recovery-based, guided self-help intervention for parents with severe mental illnesses.

Methods: Changes in the PARSS intervention group were compared with changes in a control group in a non-equivalent control group design. Outcome measures included: parenting satisfaction reported by parents; parenting success reported by mental health practitioners and family members; empowerment as reported by parents, practitioners and family members; and parents' reported quality of life. Additional process data were obtained on relationship with practitioner, quality of contact, satisfaction with the intervention and fidelity.

Results: Parenting satisfaction increased after one year for the PARSS group, but not for the control group. Parents' reports of empowerment did not change for either group. The scores of parents' empowerment reported by practitioners and family members increased in the control group, with no such change in the PARSS group. Quality of life improved significantly for the intervention group. Process measures showed that, although PARSS was not always implemented as intended, both parents and practitioners expressed satisfaction with the intervention.

Conclusions and implications for practice: The first experiences with PARSS were mixed. This intervention, implemented by mental health practitioners, has the potential to function as a useful tool for supporting parents. Attention must be paid to enhancing intervention implementation and fidelity.

3. **An interview study investigating the challenges and coping strategies of children whose parents are affected by schizophrenia which contains 34 qualitative interviews along with content analysis.**

Kahl Y & Jungbauer J (2014) Challenges and coping strategies of children with parent's affected by schizophrenia: results from an in-depth interview study. *Child and Adolescent Social Work Journal* 31 (2) 181–196.

This article presents results from an in-depth interview study investigating challenges and coping strategies of children with parents affected by schizophrenia. Thirty-four qualitative interviews of children were conducted and evaluated by content analysis. The interviewees spoke of a wide range of challenges that they must deal with daily. A variety of available coping strategies, social and personal resources were identified in the study. The results show that there is a need for professional support, especially on a low-threshold basis, that helps affected children to develop appropriate and diverse forms of coping.

4. **A study containing six semi-structured interviews with mothers in a rural mental health service in Ireland in relation to stigma and service use.**

Cremers GE, Cogan NA & Twamley I (2014) Mental health and parenting in rural areas: an exploration of parental experiences and current needs. *Journal of Mental Health* 23 (2) 99–104.

Background: Research on parental mental health problems (MHPs) has predominantly used urban samples and focused on the risks for children.

Aims: The purpose of this study was to explore rural parents' lived experiences of parenting with a MHP.

Method: Six semi-structured interviews were conducted with mothers who were using a mental health service in rural Ireland. Interpretative phenomenological analysis (IPA) was employed.

Results: Themes identified were: 'being observed and negatively judged by others'; 'overshadowed by the duality of parenting and MHPs'; 'dominance of medication over other treatment options'; 'uncertainty (of impact on parenting ability and children)' and 'need for inclusion'. Although parents' experienced a variety of concerns generic to parenting and mental health, living in a small, rural community was related to pronounced concerns regarding the stigma, devaluation and uncertainty associated with MHPs and service use.

Conclusion: Further investigation into and consideration of the specific needs and experiences of parent service-users could benefit both parents and their families and inform service development.

5. **Large research study into the service use in children of parents with recurrent depression and explores the key factors that influence such contact with services for earlier intervention strategies.**

Potter R, Mars B, Eyre O, Legge S, Ford T, Sellers R, Craddock N, Rice F, Collishaw S, Thapar A & Thapar AK (2012) Missed opportunities: mental disorder in children of parents with depression. *British Journal of General Practice* 62 (600) 360–361.

Background: Emerging evidence suggests that early intervention and prevention programmes for mental health problems in the offspring of parents with depression are important. Such programmes are difficult to implement if children with psychiatric disorders are not identified and are not accessing services, even if their parents are known to primary care.

Aim: To investigate service use in children of parents who have recurrent depression, and factors that influence such contact.

Design and setting: A total of 333 families were recruited, mainly through primary health care, in which at least one parent had received treatment for recurrent depression and had a child aged between nine and 17 years.

Method: Psychiatric assessments of parents and children were completed using research diagnostic interviews. The service-use interview recorded current (in the three months prior to interview) and lifetime contact with health, educational and social services due to concerns about the child's emotions or behaviour.

Results: Only 37% of children who met criteria for psychiatric disorder were in contact with any service at the time of interview. A third, who were suicidal or self-harming and had a psychiatric disorder at that time, were not in contact with any service. Lack of parental worry predicted lower service use, with higher rates in children with comorbidity and suicidality.

Conclusion: Most children with a psychiatric disorder in this high-risk sample were not in contact with services. Improving ease of access to services, increasing parental and professional awareness that mental health problems can cluster in families, and improving links between adult and child services may help early detection and intervention strategies for the offspring of parents with depression.

6. **Qualitative methods study exploring Community Mental Health Team (CMHT) workers' experiences of decision making in the interface between mental health and child welfare services.**

Rouf K, Larkin M & Lowe G (2012) Making decisions about parental mental health: an exploratory study of community mental health team staff. *Child Abuse Review* 21 (3) 173–189.

Adult mental health problems can impact on parents, and research shows that their children are at higher risk of developing mental health problems. In extreme cases, mental health problems are associated with a risk of fatal child abuse. Despite this, there are few studies exploring clinical decision-making by adult mental health professionals.

'In extreme cases, mental health problems are associated with a risk of fatal child abuse.'

This study used qualitative methods to explore Community Mental Health Team (CMHT) workers' experiences of decision-making in the interface between mental health and child welfare. Workers were interviewed about their experiences of clinical decision-making regarding child welfare. Interviews and accounts were analysed using Interpretative Phenomenological Analysis. Influences on decision-making were explored and triangulated with the accounts of Named Nurses for Child Protection.

The findings revealed that CMHT participants were aware of their responsibilities towards children, but a complex synthesis of factors impacted on their sense-making about risk and welfare. Three superordinate themes emerged: the tensions of working across systems; trying to balance the perceptions and feelings involved in sense-making; and the role that interpersonal dynamics play in the understanding and management of risk. This paper focuses in particular on perceptions and feelings.

Resources

Ross PDS (2015) Locating evidence for practice. In: M Webber (Ed.) *Applying Research Evidence in Social Work Practice* (pp22-43). London: Palgrave.

Useful tools and resources

Useful tools and resources

Information and resources for parents, children and families, carers and professionals

The Social Care Institute for Excellence (SCIE) parental mental health and child welfare resources

SCIE's comprehensive suite of resources includes: a review of the evidence about parental mental health and child welfare work, cross-cutting health and social care accredited guidance, e-learning, and implementation learning.
For more information visit: http://www.scie.org.uk/children/parentalmentalhealthandchildwelfare/

Wardale L (2007) Keeping the Family in Mind resource pack (2nd Edition)

For more information visit: http://www.barnardos.org.uk/keeping_family_in_mind_flyer.pdf

COPMI – children of parents with a mental illness

Mental health information and resources for Australian parents, children, families, carers and health professionals.
For more information visit: http://www.copmi.net.au

Kidstime Foundation

The foundation brings together former affected young people, nurses and psychiatrists to develop programmes aimed at promoting resilience in the children who are affected by parental mental illness and to help reduce the stigma associated with mental ill-health in general. Projects currently available at Kidstime include: 'When a Parent has a Mental Illness' film, Being Seen And Heard, The Who Cares Project, Kidstime Workshops and Working Together.
For more information visit: http://kidstimefoundation.org/current-projects-2/

The Children's Society's Engage toolkit – whole family working

The Engage toolkit brings together a range of resources to improve health and social care practice in working with and responding to the needs of the whole family.
For more information visit: http://www.engagetoolkit.org.uk/health-social-care/resources-support-whole-family-working

The Children's Society's Include programme – supporting young carers and their families

Information and resources for all professionals.
For more information visit: http://www.youngcarer.com/?file=2010102142315.htm

Mind – for better mental health

For more information visit: http://www.mind.org.uk

YoungMinds – the voice for young people's mental health and wellbeing

For more information visit: http://www.youngminds.org.uk

Services

Family Action Building Bridges

Building Bridges is Family Action's home-based family support service that works with families with multiple complex needs in order to make families stronger, safer and more fulfilling for children and parents. Building Bridges works with families that might have problems such as parental mental health, a young carer at home, difficulties in parenting, children with mental health or behavioural difficulties, relationship issues, safeguarding issues and financial and material hardship. They work with families to:

- promote good health
- meet emotional needs
- keep children safe
- feel part of their community
- support learning
- set boundaries
- encourage work aspirations
- provide a stable home
- manage their finances

For more information, visit: https://www.family-action.org.uk/building-bridges/

Anna Freud Centre – The Early Years Parenting Unit (EYPU)

The Early Years Parenting Unit (EYPU) is a specialist service offering assessment and therapy for parents with personality disorders/difficulties with babies and children under the age of five who are subject to a Child in Need or Child Protection plan, or who are on the edge of care.
For more information visit: http://www.annafreud.org/services-schools/services-for-parents/early-years-parenting-unit/

The Early Years Parenting Unit: A developing manual of practice and service set-up

This manual provides you with a step-by-step guide to setting up your own Early Years Parenting Unit (EYPU). The Unit is based on an approach called mentalisation-based practice. Working in collaboration with children's social care is fundamental to its effectiveness. The manual will introduce to why EYPUs are needed, the therapeutic day programme at EYPU and the difference that it makes to families where parents are experiencing personality disorder/difficulties.

Who is this manual for?

This manual is for anyone interested in setting up their own early years parenting programme. It is for primarily for workers but it is OPEN SOURCE so that if service users or other parties are interested they are welcome to look and contribute their feedback too.

The following groups will find the manual most useful:

- Social workers
- Clinical psychologists
- Adult and child psychiatrists
- Family therapists
- Children and adolescent mental health service (CAMHS) workers
- Health and social care commissioners.

Benefits of using the manual

The manual will benefit your practice by:

- providing you with a detailed guide to setting up your own EYPU that can be adapted to your own local circumstances
- demonstrating how EYPU's approach to jointly managing cases with children's social care results in more effective management and timely decision-making in relation to complex, high-risk families
- introducing you to mentalisation-based practice and the difference that it can make to families where parents are experiencing personality disorder/difficulties.

For more information, visit: http://eypu.tiddlyspace.com/

NSPCC – Family SMILES – supporting children living with parents with mental health issues

Family SMILES aims to help children aged eight to 14 years old to build self-esteem, resilience and life skills. Family SMILES also works with parents to help them understand the impact of their illness on their child and to improve their parenting skills to provide a safe, secure and supportive family environment.

For more information visit: http://www.nspcc.org.uk/services-and-resources/services-for-children-and-families/family-smiles/

Young Carers Research Group – Loughborough University

Downloadable publications, resources, current research, young carers' needs analysis, publications and young carers' mental health.
For more information visit: http://www.lboro.ac.uk/microsites/socialsciences/ycrg/

Carers UK – making life better for carers

For more information visit: http://www.carersuk.org/help-and-advice

Carers Trust – action, help, advice

For more information visit: www.carers.org.uk

Carers Trust, whole family approach – practice examples

This is a collection of practice examples to support those who commission or develop services to think about how to deliver creative and effective services locally.
For more information visit: https://professionals.carers.org/whole-family-approach-practice-examples

Assessment, planning and prevention

Interface – schools. Vulnerable children audit tool

Interface have worked with schools to develop an electronic tool to help school leaders, governors, teachers, support staff and multi-agency partners to identify vulnerable children and their families and work more effectively with them.
For more information visit: http://www.interfaceenterprises.co.uk/consultancy/schools-vulnerable-children-audit-tool/

The Young Carers Research Group Loughborough

Identifying and recognising the needs of young carers – new mental health questionnaire and screening tool

The Young Carers Research Group has launched a new questionnaire and screening tool to help researchers and health, social care and education professionals estimate the prevalence of young carers in a given area and to identify their needs. The YC-QST-20 (mental health) is intended to be used as a research and screening tool among children who may be living with, and/or caring for, a relative in the home (such as a parent, grandparent or sibling) with a mental health problem/mental illness. The YC-QST-20 is also intended to gauge children's level of understanding about their relative's illness/mental health problem, the nature and extent of children's caring responsibilities and their needs as carers.

To access the YC-QST-20 (mental health) and the explanatory model, go to http://www.lboro.ac.uk/microsites/socialsciences/ycrg/resources.html

Message in a Bottle – Barnardo's Action with Young Carers Liverpool

The Message in a Bottle Pack (the pot was adapted with kind permission from the Lions) designed in partnership with families, helps people to think and prepare for any medical and family emergencies, relieving many of the concerns that young carers have including thinking they are responsible for their parent's ill health. Together, an advance statement and message in a bottle support plan can help to support the whole family.

For further information contact: Louise Wardale, Keeping the Family in Mind Co-ordinator, Barnardo's Action with Young Carers Liverpool. Email: louise.wardale@barnardos.org.uk

Promoting family contact when a parent is in hospital

Mersey Care NHS Trust and Barnardo's family rooms – family rooms for young carers visiting relatives using inpatient mental health services

Mersey Care NHS Trust runs this service in partnership with Barnardo's Keeping the Family in Mind (KFIM) – a project to engage young carers in the delivery of services for families affected by mental health issues. This is part of the Barnardo's Action with Young Carers (AWYC) service in Liverpool.

Family rooms provide a safe, comfortable and homely environment for children, young people and their families when they visit a family member staying in a specialist mental health, learning disability or substance misuse service. The family rooms have all been designed with young carers to make sure they are in an environment which is a home away from home. The services have been running since 2001.

For further information contact: Carol Bernard, Director of Commissioning, Mersey Care NHS Trust.
Email: carol.bernard@merseycare.nhs.uk or

Louise Wardale, Keeping the Family in Mind Co-ordinator, Barnardo's Action with Young Carers Liverpool.
Email: louise.wardale@barnardos.org.uk

Also see: https://professionals.carers.org/sites/default/files/liverpool-famroomslinks-proof2-6568.pdf

Mersey Care NHS Trust – thinking family in high secure services

Think Family is showcased in a film produced by Secure Services Division for family visiting arrangements at Ashworth Hospital Mersey Care NHS Trust – web reference to view an online film for families and children can be found at: http://www.merseycare.nhs.uk/contact-us/media-centre/our-films/bringing-children-to-ashworth-hospital/

Leaflets and factsheets

The Royal College of Psychiatrists

Mental health and growing up factsheet

Parental mental illness, the impact on children and adolescents: information for parents, carers and anyone who works with young people.
For more information visit: http://www.rcpsych.ac.uk/healthadvice/parentsandyouthinfo/parentscarers/parentalmentalillness.aspx

Parents and youth info index

This index provides specifically tailored information for young people, parents, teachers and carers about mental health.
For more information visit: http://www.rcpsych.ac.uk/healthadvice/parentsandyouthinfo.aspx

Mental health and growing up

Factsheets for parents, teachers and young people.
For more information visit: http://www.rcpsych.ac.uk/usefulresources/publications/books/rcpp/9781908020468.aspx

So your Mum or Dad has a mental illness – leaflets for children and young people

Children and Young People's Strategic Partnership (CYPSP) Northern Ireland & Participation Network - supporting the public sector to engage with children and young people.
For more information visit: http://www.cypsp.org/wp-content/uploads/2014/08/Think_Family_Leaflet_Childrens.pdf
http://www.cypsp.org/wp-content/uploads/2014/08/Think_Family_Leaflet_Young_People_%282%29.pdf

Training and workforce development

The Family Model – an integrated approach to support mentally ill parents and their children

For more information visit: http://www.thefamilymodel.com

The Centre for Parent and Child Support and The Family Partnership Model – South London and Maudsley NHS Foundation Trust

For more information visit: http://www.cpcs.org.uk

Interface

Interface is a national provider of specialist support, training, information and resources for those working to transform the lives of vulnerable families. Interface's aim is to enhance capacity and expertise in local areas and we do this across priority areas of service delivery for communities, children and vulnerable families.
For more information visit: http://www.interfaceenterprises.co.uk/about-us/

The Meriden Family Programme – NHS

For more information visit: http://www.meridenfamilyprogramme.com

Anna Freud Centre – training and research

For more information visit: http://www.annafreud.org/training-research/training-and-conferences-overview/

SCIE e-Learning – parental mental health and families

For more information visit: http://www.scie.org.uk/publications/elearning/parental mentalhealthandfamilies/index.asp

SCIE parental mental health and child welfare videos on Social Care TV

There are three SCIE videos on Social Care TV about parental mental health and child welfare:

- ▶ 'The Practitioners' Perspective' – a film about professional perspectives on working with parents with mental health problems and their children
- ▶ 'A Young Person's Story' – a film about a young carer's experience of trying to get the support she needed
- ▶ 'A Mother's Story' – a film about a mother's experience of getting the support she needed for herself and her family

For more information visit: http://www.scie.org.uk/socialcaretv/topic.asp?t=parentalmentalhealthandchildwelfare

The Royal College of Psychiatrists film. 'When a parent has a mental illness – on coping with a parent with a mental illness'

For more information visit: http://www.rcpsych.ac.uk/healthadvice/parentsandyouthinfo/youngpeople/caringforaparent.aspx

Policy and practice guidance

No Wrong Doors: Working together to support young carers and their families

A template for a local memorandum of understanding between statutory directors for children's and adult services – March 2015.
For more information visit: http://www.local.gov.uk/documents/10180/11431/No+wrong+doors+-+working+together+to+support+young+carers+and+their+families/d210a4a6-b352-4776-b858-f3adf06e4b66

SCIE – The Care Act: Transition from childhood to adulthood (2015)

For more information visit: http://www.scie.org.uk/care-act-2014/transition-from-childhood-to-adulthood/

SCIE (2015) – Transition from children's to adult services – early and comprehensive identification

For more information visit: http://www.scie.org.uk/care-act-2014/transition-from-childhood-to-adulthood/early-comprehensive-identification/index.asp

SCIE (2015) Young carer transition in practice under the Care Act 2014

For more information visit: http://www.scie.org.uk/care-act-2014/transition-from-childhood-to-adulthood/young-carer-transition-in-practice/index.asp

SCIE Accredited Guide 30 (updated 2011). Think Child, Think Parent, Think Family: A guide to parental mental health and child welfare

This guide has not been updated since December 2011. It may not reflect current policy but still provides valuable practice guidance.
For more information visit: http://www.scie.org.uk/publications/guides/guide30/index.asp

Falkov A (2014) The Children of Parents with a Mental Illness (COPMI) GEMS – The Continuum of Need: Parental mental health is everyone's responsibility

The 'Continuum of Need' provides a basis for thinking about levels of need along a theoretical continuum, based on the diversity of individuals' needs within families.
For more information visit: http://www.copmi.net.au/images/pdf/Research/gems-edition-17-may-2014.pdf

Keeping the Family in Mind: A briefing on young carers whose parents have mental health problems (2005)

For more information visit: http://www.barnardos.org.uk/keeping_the_family_in_mind.pdf

Research

Family Potential

The focus of the Family Potential Research Centre is to develop innovative ways of thinking that cut across traditional domains of services and renegotiate traditional child/parent focused policy and practice. The research centre is responding to the dearth of research looking at a genuinely 'whole family' perspective. Through understanding the lived experience of families, the research centre aims to develop service models, inform professional practice and influence policy to enable strategies to develop and flourish that mobilise family strengths and potential.
For more information visit: http://www.familypotential.org

Family Potential – Centre for Policy and Practice Research – Knowledge Exchange

The Knowledge Exchange hosts summaries of innovative or interesting work that organisations are doing using a 'whole family' or 'think family' approach.
For more information visit: http://www.familypotential.org/?page_id=318

COPMI Gems research summaries – Gateways to Evidence that Matters

The aim of the Gateways to Evidence that Matters (GEMS) is to provide a summary of recent Australian and international research concerning children (aged 0-18 years) of parents with a mental illness, their parents and families. While research in this area is growing, there is a lack of evidence-based practice when working with families affected by parental mental illness.

These GEMS have been prepared as a resource for those working in the field, and aim to provide a synthesis of available research that might guide and direct practitioners, and highlight current research and practice gaps.

GEMS promotes the collection, interpretation and integration of valid, recent and relevant research from around the world, based on the views and experiences of those researching, working and living with parental mental illness.

For more information visit: http://www.copmi.net.au/professionals-organisations/what-works/research-summaries-gems

Your Family, Your Voice: An alliance of families and practitioners working to transform the system

Your Family, Your Voice: An Alliance of families and practitioners working to transform the system (formerly working title the Struggling Families Alliance) is a three-year programme of work that began in June 2014. It is led by Family Rights Group with empirical research conducted by professors Brigid Featherstone and Kate Morris.

The Alliance will work:

▶ to counter the stigma, negative presumptions and judgemental approaches to families whose children are subject to, or at risk of, state intervention, by influencing how these families are perceived by the public and portrayed by the media and politicians

▶ to influence law, policy, practice and service design and delivery so that our child welfare, child mental health, youth justice and education systems promote effective human functioning and healthy relationships

▶ to enable these families to have a voice in policy and decision-making circles.

For more information, visit: http://www.frg.org.uk/involving-families/your-family,-your-voice

Related publications

Parental Psychiatric Disorder: Distressed parents and their families (3rd Edition)

Parental Psychiatric Disorder presents an innovative approach to thinking about and working with families where a parent has a mental illness. With 30 new chapters from an internationally renowned author team, this new edition presents the current state of knowledge in this critically important field. Issues around prevalence, stigma and systems theory provide a foundation for the book, which offers new paradigms for understanding mental illness in families. The impact of various parental psychiatric disorders on children and family relationships are summarised, including coverage of schizophrenia, depression, anxiety, substance abuse disorders, eating disorders, personality disorders and trauma. Multiple innovative interventions are outlined, targeting children, parents and families, as well as strategies that foster workforce and organisational development. Incorporating different theoretical frameworks, the book enhances understanding of the dimensions of psychiatric disorders from a multigenerational perspective, making this an invaluable text for students, researchers and clinicians from many mental health disciplines.

Reupert A, Maybery D, Nicholson J, Gopfert M & Seeman M (2015) *Parental Psychiatric Disorder – Distressed Parents and their Families* (3rd Edition). Cambridge: Cambridge University Press.

Think Family: Progress report

For more information visit: http://www.merseycare.nhs.uk/media/1065/think-family-progress-report-final-version.pdf

Butterworth J (JMB Health Consultancy) (2014) Think Family – Progress Report: Liverpool Barnardo's.

Out of the Mainstream: Helping the children of parents with a mental illness

Out of the Mainstream considers how the diverse groups of agencies, specialist teams and groups in the community can work together, even when many barriers may hinder the effective co-working between individuals and these various groups. It is an invaluable resource for psychologists, psychiatrists, social workers, health visitors, mental health nurses, teachers and voluntary sector agency staff.

Loshak R (2013) *Out of the Mainstream – Helping the children of parents with a mental illness*. London: Routledge.

Parents as patients: Supporting the needs of patients who are parents and their children

For more information visit: http://www.rcpsych.ac.uk/usefulresources/publications/collegereports/cr/cr164.aspx

Royal College of Psychiatrists (2010) CR164. Parents as patients: Supporting the needs of patients who are parents and their children.

Parents in Hospital: How mental health services can best promote family contact when a parent is in hospital

For more information visit: http://www.barnardos.org.uk/resources/research_and_publications/parents-in-hospital-how-mental-health-services-can-best-promote-family-contact-when-a-parent-is-in-hospital/publication-view.jsp?pid=PUB-1393

Robinson B & Scott S (2007) *Parents in Hospital: How mental health services can best promote family contact when a parent is in hospital*. Barnardo's.

Resources from Pavilion

The Family Model Handbook: An integrated approach to supporting mentally ill parents and their children

This presents The Family Model approach to working with parental mental illness and effects on family relationships, children's needs and parenting, for clinicians and managers.

For more information visit: www.pavpub.com/the-family-model-handbook/

Falkov A (2013) *The Family Model Handbook: An integrated approach to supporting mentally ill parents and their children.* Brighton: Pavilion Publishing.

Attachment-based Practice with Adults

For more information visit: www.pavpub.com/attachment-based-practice-with-adults/

Baim C & Morrison T (2011) *Attachment-based Practice with Adults.* Brighton: Pavilion Publishing.

Bipolar Disorder: A guide for mental health professionals and those who live with it

For more information visit: www.pavpub.com/bipolar-disorder/

Walsh D & Smith R (2012) *Bipolar Disorder: A guide for mental health professionals and those who live with it.* Brighton: Pavilion Publishing.

Assessment and Management of Risk in Child Care and Child Protection

For more information visit: www.pavpub.com/assessment-and-management-of-risk-in-child-care-and-child-protection/

Risk Decision Making: Working with risk and implementing positive risk taking

For more information visit: www.pavpub.com/risk-decision-making/

Forthcoming

Participatory Research: Working with vulnerable groups in research and practice

Jo Aldridge's new book, *Participatory research: Working with vulnerable groups in research and practice*, to be published by The Policy Press, includes in-depth case studies and examples of participatory research methods that have been used with young carers and their families, as well as with people with profound learning difficulties and unsupported women victims of domestic violence. The book also includes a new participatory research model that provides researchers, academics and students with clear parameters for working more effectively with vulnerable or marginalised groups. The book includes extensive discussion and examination of what is meant by 'vulnerability' in different health, social care and academic contexts, as well as from the perspectives of people defined as 'vulnerable' themselves. More details about the book, including ordering information, can be found at: http://www.lboro.ac.uk/microsites/socialsciences/ycrg/youngCarersDownload/NTI_Aldridge.pdf

Aldridge J (2016) *Participatory Research: Working with vulnerable groups in research and practice.* Policy Press.